ME/CFS and
Long Covid

ME/CFS and Long Covid

Diagnosis and management of chronic fatigue syndromes

Gavin Spickett

Retired Consultant in Immunology, Allergy & General Medicine

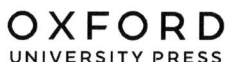

OXFORD
UNIVERSITY PRESS

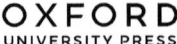

OXFORD
UNIVERSITY PRESS

Great Clarendon Street, Oxford, OX2 6DP,
United Kingdom

Oxford University Press is a department of the University of Oxford.
It furthers the University's objective of excellence in research, scholarship,
and education by publishing worldwide. Oxford is a registered trade mark of
Oxford University Press in the UK and in certain other countries.

© Oxford University Press 2025

The moral rights of the author have been asserted.

Published in the United States of America by Oxford University Press
198 Madison Avenue, New York, NY 10016, United States of America.

British Library Cataloguing in Publication Data

Data available

Library of Congress Control Number: 2025933829

ISBN 978–0–19–896213–7

DOI: 10.1093/med/9780198962137.001.0001

Printed and bound by
CPI Group (UK) Ltd., Croydon, CR0 4YY

Oxford University Press makes no representation, express or implied, that the
drug dosages in this book are correct. Readers must therefore always check
the product information and clinical procedures with the most up-to-date
published product information and data sheets provided by the manufacturers
and the most recent codes of conduct and safety regulations. The authors and
the publishers do not accept responsibility or legal liability for any errors in the
text or for the misuse or misapplication of material in this work. Except where
otherwise stated, drug dosages and recommendations are for the non-pregnant
adult who is not breast-feeding.

The manufacturer's authorised representative in the EU for product safety is Oxford
University Press España S.A. of El Parque Empresarial San Fernando de Henares,
Avenida de Castilla, 2 – 28830 Madrid (www.oup.es/en or product.safety@oup.
com). OUP España S.A. also acts as importer into Spain of products made by the
manufacturer.

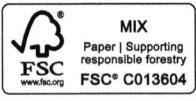

Preface

This book is aimed primarily at non-specialist doctors and other healthcare professionals who encounter chronic fatigue syndrome, also known as ME or ME/CFS (myalgic encephalomyelitis) and the post-Covid variant called Long Covid (but in reality, another version of post-infectious chronic fatigue). It may be of interest to some patients who want to read more about their condition.

It is the distillation of what I have learned and unlearned over the course of a career diagnosing and managing patients referred to me with suspected chronic fatigue syndrome. On a rough calculation, I have seen over 3,000 new patients with fatigue. Over the course of my career, I have worked with a range of therapists and other medical specialists and learned about areas of medicine, such as sleep disorders and how to recognize them, that I never expected to be involved in when I started my career in Immunology. I have had a lot of support from other physicians in this learning process, but I have learned even more from my discussions with my patients. I make no apology that this little book is sprinkled with personal observations, based on what I have learned from my patients and my colleagues.

Over my career I have seen ME/CFS move from a despised non-illness to a more widely accepted physical illness that is not just laziness or wilful manipulation of the benefits system. However not all doctors or healthcare workers have yet taken on board the messages coming from current research and from professional bodies. The biggest change has been that we are now seeing properly conducted research being supported, for example by the Medical Research Council in the UK, the European Network and the Institute of Medicine in the USA, and this is at last leading to significant insights into the pathogenesis of the illness, although not yet to major breakthroughs in treatment. This is no less than sufferers deserve.

The biggest breakthrough though is a consequence of the COVID-19 pandemic. When the pandemic first started, my immediate reaction was, 'Oh no, this is going to cause a huge surge in cases of chronic fatigue syndrome'. It did, although it has been given a special and entirely unwarranted new name ('Long Covid'). This is essentially a severe post-infectious chronic fatigue syndrome and the symptomatology of Long Covid is pretty much identical to ME/CFS, with the exception of oddities specific to COVID-19 infection such as anosmia (due to the virus binding via ACE2 receptors on olfactory cells in the nose). Some of the differences are down to the fact that 'Long Covid' patients are being seen much earlier in their illness, allowing us to look at early pathology that we have rarely or never seen in patients with ME/CFS, because the patients are referred too late. It has been known for many years that infections can trigger ME/CFS. Because Long Covid has affected a significant number of doctors and other healthcare workers, the medical profession has to differentiate it from ME/CFS, because, still, many doctors and healthcare workers are conditioned to think that ME/CFS is a psychological not medical illness and they couldn't possibly have a psychological illness. However you classify it, the development of Long Covid has at last led to some high grade clinical and scientific research, which is already leading to a greater understanding of the mechanisms involved in causing chronic fatigue not just in Long Covid but other chronic fatigue syndromes including ME/CFS and post-viral fatigue syndromes. Hopefully this surge in research will lead to new and different approaches to treatment. Everything now points to neuroinflammation, triggered by the immune response to viral infection.

All the patients who have been to see me want some straightforward things. Most, by the time I see them, have been ill for some time and have done their own research through Dr Google. They know that there is unlikely to be a magic cure. What they seek above all is to meet a doctor who will sit and listen properly to their story, assess them competently, and give them answers to entirely reasonable questions and provide them with advice and support to help them adjust to their 'new normal', to purloin a phrase from the COVID-19 crisis. What is not helpful is for doctors and healthcare workers to brush off their symptoms, tell them it's all in the mind, tell them they are simply depressed, tell them to pull their socks up, tell them to go out and do unstructured exercise and to provide no practical help with symptoms management. I do not view these desires as inappropriate or unreasonable.

One of the biggest problems for patients is the need for legitimacy. This means that ME/CFS and Long Covid must be accepted as real illnesses. They are not just 'medically unexplained symptoms': we know enough now about the science of ME/CFS to realize that this is as unjustified as referring to the illness as 'yuppy flu'. Medicine has a peculiarly repulsive habit of blaming the patients as 'mad' or 'bad' whenever there is no immediate explanation for symptoms. I always use the example of gastric ulcers: at the end of the nineteenth and beginning of the twentieth century this condition was thought to be due to psychological weaknesses in the sufferer. Of course, someone who has chronic pain from their chronic stomach ulcer is going to feel psychologically disturbed—but that is not the cause of the ulcer. By the end of the twentieth century we knew that gastric ulcers are caused by a bacterium called *Helicobacter pylori*, which is readily treatable with acid suppression therapy plus combination antibiotics. Now, no one would dream of suggesting that gastric ulcers are caused by psychological weakness. Exactly the same reasoning applies to someone suffering in the twenty-first century from ME/CFS: doctors must not assume that the patient is mad or bad just because they and the treating doctor do not understand the cause of the illness. Unfortunately, despite the upsurge in knowledge and the recognition by major health bodies that ME/CFS and Long Covid) are real medical illnesses not psychological or psychiatric illnesses, there are still headlines in 2024 about appalling treatment of ME/CFS sufferers by non-specialists in UK hospitals: *https://www.*

bbc.co.uk/news/articles/c9rry6lr54lo   and   *https://www.bbc.co.uk/news/articles/ c2q03ppzzzOo* which show that there still a huge uphill struggle to ensure that the latest knowledge about ME/CFS and Long Covid reaches those who provide care to patients. Another case from 2024 highlights the unimaginably severe impact that ME/CFS can have on people, leading them to seek assisted suicide (*https:// www.bbc.co.uk/news/articles/c51y7zq4pgno*). This book provides the basic knowledge to do this effectively.

This book does not pretend to have all the answers. Its primary purposes are to encourage healthcare professionals to care for their ME/CFS and Long Covid patients in a humane and empathic way, acknowledging the limitations of our knowledge at present but offering suitable support and encouragement. There will be a medical/physiological explanation forthcoming and I am sure that it will be a surprise to many and a great shock to some. There will be treatments in the future and doctors in 10–20 years' time will look back at what was done to ME/CFS patients today with the same horror that we look back at some of the treatments offered in the name of medicine for common conditions in the nineteenth and early twentieth centuries. This book does not give details of the mass of often conflicting and impenetrable research on fatigue, much of which has yet to be confirmed and integrated into a clear scientific overview of the cause of 'chronic fatigue'. Where possible, I have selected interesting and pertinent references for each subsection as further reading, but this book is about practical management and is not about citing all possible references! Because of the rapidity of advancing science, even these references may be out of date by the time the book is published. The reader is therefore advised to use a reputable search engine for scientific literature, such as PubMed or Google Scholar, to check for the most up-to-date information.

As a caution, I would draw attention to journals, especially special editions published by the Hindawi Brand, bought out by John Wiley in 2021. Investigations have led to the suspension of a number of journals in this brand and large-scale retractions of papers by John Wiley, on suspicions that there has been large-scale use of paper mills and fraudulent behaviour by some guest editors (*https:// www.wiley.com/en-us/network/publishing/research-publishing/open-access/address ing-paper-mills-and-a-way-forward-for-journal-security*). This process is still ongoing. It is clear that John Wiley journals are not the only ones affected. Some journal websites have been hacked to redirect submissions to cloned websites where fraudulent papers, often AI produced, are published electronically. Some of the references in this book may be affected, so caution is advised before reliance is placed on cited references, as some may be subject to withdrawal.

It must be stressed that chronic fatigue is not just about ME/CFS and Long Covid. Chronic fatigue is an integral part of almost all chronic illnesses, which is why very careful assessment is required to ensure that medical treatable conditions associated with chronic fatigue are diagnosed and treated. Conditions other than ME/CFS and Long Covid may account for nearly half of all referrals to a chronic fatigue clinic, from my analysis of my own referral practice. As well as managing the underlying conditions that cause fatigue, it is important to manage the fatigue too. Many of the principles of management that are applicable to ME/CFS and Long Covid are applicable to chronic fatigue of other causes. This book therefore is about more than just ME/CFS and Long Covid.

Acknowledgements

This book would not have been possible without the learning opportunities created by my patients. Learning medicine from books, papers, colleagues, and lectures only provides a skeleton. The flesh is provided by dealing directly with patients and spending enough time talking to them to hear and understand their stories. So, my primary dedication is to my patients.

I never really set out in my career to develop an interest ME/CFS, but the patients just came and in the early 1990s there were few places that they could go. I could not turn them away. There were patient groups desperately struggling to get recognition for the condition and I record the debt that current patients owe to these pioneers who persuaded the chief medical officers to start taking the illness seriously, which eventually led to direct NHS funding to set up specialist diagnostic and therapy services (in England) and eventually to NICE guidelines, recognizing that these proved contentious at the time and even now. Our own services in Newcastle owed a lot to Dr Mike Snow, an infectious disease consultant, who, through his own clinical practice, helped develop not only our local services but also our Region-wide network. He guided and advised me in my early career as a consultant with an interest in ME/CFS.

I also acknowledge the help of the therapists who were recruited to the fledging services in the North-East and North Cumbria, some of whom are still working in the field 15 years on. It is invidious to pick names as all of them have contributed to my own knowledge and understanding, through the multidisciplinary framework that was established. We were able to recruit a very able Regional Network co-ordinator, Louise Wilson, and administrator Jill Bullimore. It has been a pleasure to work with all of them.

My clinical colleagues in Newcastle have been a profound source of knowledge and expertise that I could call on for help and advice. I shared the ME/CFS load with my colleagues in the Department of Infectious Diseases until I retired, when they shouldered the whole burden. I am particularly grateful to Dr Kirsty Anderson, consultant neurologist, who educated me about sleep disorders and how to recognize them, and Dr Andy James, consultant endocrinologist, who was always willing to advise about any suspected endocrine problem. It was stimulating to be able to discuss fatigue with my academic colleague, Professor Julia Newton, officially a consultant geriatrician, but actually an academic expert in the mechanisms of fatigue. She recognized that there are other causes of chronic fatigue apart from ME/CFS and set up a clinic for these patients too.

Working in the field of ME/CFS has been challenging but enjoyable. Every patient was a new detective challenge to work out whether there was any other cause for the fatigue. I have always enjoyed 'general medicine', and chronic fatigue ensured that I kept my generalist skills up to scratch.

Of course, I also owe a debt to my wife Sally for putting up with my long hours, setting off early for outreach chronic fatigue clinics in Keswick and arriving back late, and also for putting up with my study littered with books and papers. I am extremely grateful to the editorial team at OUP for their help with this project.

Thank you all.

Contents

About the author

Dr Gavin Spickett is a retired consultant in immunology, allergy, and general medicine. He trained in medicine at the University of Oxford and earned his DPhil at the MRC Cellular Immunology Unit, Oxford. He completed general medical training in Ipswich and trained in immunology, allergy, and immunopathology at the MRC Clinical Research Centre, Harrow, and the Department of Immunology at the John Radcliffe Hospital, Oxford. In 1991, he took up the position of consultant clinical immunologist, allergist, and general physician in Newcastle, where he worked until retirement in 2021. During his career, he developed the Regional Clinical Immunology and Allergy service and the associated laboratory service. He established and led the Regional Chronic Fatigue Network and was the lead clinician for ME/CFS at the Royal Victoria Infirmary. In 2017, he was awarded a Lifetime Achievement Award by the UK Primary Immunodeficiency Network for his work for patients with primary immunodeficiencies.

CHAPTER 1

The history of chronic fatigue syndromes including ME/CFS and Long Covid

> **KEY POINTS**
>
> * ME/CFS is not a new illness, having been clearly described in the mid-19th century.
> * Lack of understanding of the cause has led to misclassification as a psychiatric/psychological disease.
> * There have been many outbreaks of ME/CFS throughout the twentieth century, although no clear infective agents were described. Sporadic cases of ME/CFS predominated during the late twentieth and early twenty-first centuries.
> * Application of modern diagnostic tools has been able to link chronic fatigue with MERS and SARS infections and, more recently, Long Covid with SARS-CoV2.
> * There is now recognition that ME/CFS symptoms may be seen after the common cold.
> * There has been progressive recognition by major national health bodies in the USA, UK, and elsewhere that ME/CFS (and Long Covid) represent chronic medical conditions.

1.1 The origins and history of chronic fatigue

It is widely perceived that ME/CFS is a new disease. It is not. Romantic literature of the eighteenth century contains descriptions of people, mainly women, with symptoms that we would recognize today as chronic fatigue. The caveat is that at this time there were other chronic illnesses that would also cause chronic fatigue, such as tuberculosis, which were not recognized. This makes definitive retrospective diagnosis impossible.

The first distinctive recognition of a CFS-like illness was in the mid-nineteenth century. An American doctor, George Miller Beard, who served as an assistant surgeon in the US Navy in the American Civil War, described the condition of neurasthenia. This constellation was for a long time referred to as Beard's disease. The term is no longer used. This illness was characterized by the following symptoms:

Fatigue
Anxiety and depression

Headache
Impotence
Neuralgia
Exhaustion of the nervous system's energy resources
Associated with the 'stress of urbanization' (this was the nineteenth century!)

This was a remarkably accurate description for the time of what we would now recognize as ME/CFS. The concept of neurasthenia remained popular well into the early twentieth century and other similar syndromes were described such as 'Effort syndrome' and 'Da Costa's syndrome' which are almost certainly slightly different manifestations of the same condition. As time passed, it was thought that these conditions were largely behavioural and neurasthenia was categorized in the ICD-10 classification of disease as F48—other neurotic disorders! ICD-11 has removed this label! Chronic fatigue syndrome itself has had a chequered classification career. In ICD-9 it was classified under Fatigue (780.71); in ICD-10, it moved to Disease of the Nervous System (Other disorders) as G93.32 (post-viral fatigue was G93.32). In ICD-11, it is classified under Other Disorders of the nervous system as 8E49, excluding other types of fatigue (MG22). This migration reflects the changing perceptions of the illness.

Between 1915 and 1926, there was a worldwide pandemic of 'encephalitis lethargica'. This was around the same time as the global flu epidemic, which was certainly complicated by encephalitis and parkinsonian features. However, the link between encephalitis lethargic and influenza has been questioned. In 2012, a retrospective investigation identified an enterovirus in pathological material from cases of encephalitis lethargica (Dourmashkin et al 2012). More than a million people are estimated to have been affected and some 500,000 are thought to have died. Survivors never recovered completely. The disease ceased around 1927. Historically cases of febrile illnesses complicated by lethargy and parkinsonian features have been documented back as far as 1580, with further reports at regular intervals through the centuries. These episodes sound suspiciously like a very severe post-infectious chronic fatigue, triggered by a pandemic infection, and with specific parkinsonian features (rare in ME/CFS today). There are significant parallels between the SARS-CoV2 pandemic and Long Covid.

In the 1930s there were a number of outbreaks of a chronic fatigue illness, which at the time were attributed to abortive poliovirus infection, there being no effective polio vaccine until the development of the Salk vaccine in 1952. These included the Wisconsin Convent Disease at St. Agnes Convent in 1936, an outbreak of 'abortive polio' in Swiss Towns and Army in 1937–39 and a polio-like illness in 1934 in Los Angeles. These episodes continued to be reported through to the 1980s, but have subsequently petered out.[1] This illustrates a curious pattern of illness in ME/CFS. Early cases all seem to be in localized (recognized?)

---

[1] See Me-Pedia, https://me-pedia.org/wiki/List_of_myalgic_encephalomyelitis_and_chronic_fatigue_syndrome_outbreaks

geographic clusters, whereas from the 1990s onwards, up until MERS, SARS, and SARs-CoV2, cases seem to have become more generally and randomly distributed. Why this change has occurred is unclear.

Some of the outbreaks involved significant numbers of affected people and some achieved significant public and scientific recognition. There were two major outbreaks in Iceland in 1946–47 and again in 1948–49 (Akureyri or Icelandic Disease), Adelaide in 1949–53, and the Royal Free Hospital outbreak, affecting hospital staff in 1955. The latter was extensively investigated at the time and in subsequent follow-up studies. A retrospective review in 2020 by Underhill & Baillod suggested that the McEvedy & Beard hypothesis of 1970 that it was due to mass hysteria was not true, on the basis of the very distant recollections of staff who were present in 1955, and that the significant biochemical and haematological abnormalities and evidence of brain and spinal cord inflammation (which led to the name of myalgic encephalomyelitis) were ignored, and which would be entirely inconsistent with a psychosomatic cause. Attempts to retrospectively attribute a psychosomatic cause to the Royal Free Outbreak demonstrates a persistent desire by some people to shoe-horn ME/CFS into the box labelled 'psychosomatic' irrespective of other evidence of organic disease. This has hampered high-quality research. A symposium at the Royal Society of Medicine in 1978 concluded that epidemic myalgic encephalomyelitis was a distinct disease entity. A neuroimmune cause was presciently suggested. The influence of the McEvedy and Beard hypothesis led to generations of patients being labelled as having psychosomatic illness and effectively being denied access to clinical support, as well as preventing research that would have led to earlier identification of the real pathology. In 1997 Elaine Showalter described ME/CFS as a 'hysterical narrative', a modern manifestation of hysteria, a self-perpetuating 'cultural symptom of anxiety and stress', which reinforced the marginalization of these patients.

Attempts to identify causative organisms in these early outbreaks were limited by the available diagnostic tools. Poliovirus was blamed for a number of the early pre-WWII outbreaks. In the 1960s in the USA, Epstein–Barr virus (EBV) was a favoured cause. However, this attribution was flawed for two main reasons: firstly, EBV is a ubiquitous infection, with most people having evidence of previous infection (detected by serology, the detection of antibodies to the virus) by their early 20s, so any cases of chronic fatigue in adults were likely to show evidence of previous EBV infection; secondly, benefit rules in the USA in the 1960s required people claiming benefits for ME/CFS to have serological evidence of past EBV, thus creating a circular argument about EBV causing ME/CFS!, as ME/CFS could only be diagnosed if EBV antibodies were present!

The occurrence of epidemic ME/CFS has always strongly suggested that at least in the epidemic, if not the sporadic form, the illness is triggered as a consequence of infection. The outbreak of swine flu in 2009 was accompanied by a slight increase in cases of post-infectious CFS, mainly in young people, but the prompt introduction of widespread vaccination and possibly the use of antivirals mitigated the effects. In most outbreaks, up until SARS-CoV2, however, a clear-cut association with an identified infectious agent has not been proven. There were however a small number of cases of post-infectious fatigue following the outbreaks of MERS and SARS, but as the total case numbers for these infections were small, the impact was minimal. It is for this reason that COVID-19 has been so valuable as there is a huge worldwide cohort of people who have had repeated COVID-19 antigen and antibody tests and their illness can be followed over a long time scale. The impact of vaccination can also be assessed. The most recent research has shown that other respiratory viral infections such as the common cold may also be associated with persistent fatigue symptoms. Intercurrent infections in people with existing ME/CFS and Long Covid invariably cause flares of the illness.

For a number of years in the 1980s and 1990s, Coxsackieviruses were thought to be a causative organism for ME/CFS. Coxsackieviruses are a similar type of viruses to polioviruses. Another related virus group are the Echoviruses, which are known to causes a severe and persistent illness in patients with underlying immune deficiencies. All of these viruses are grouped within the larger group of enteroviruses. Convincing evidence that enteroviruses are a major cause of ME/CFS is lacking. Some of the early studies were based on testing for VP1 antigen, but the testing was later discredited. Chronic infection with enteroviruses was suggested as a cause of ME/CFS, although it is rare for this class of viruses to cause chronic infection except in immunodeficient patients (specifically X-linked agammaglobulinaemia). There is no evidence that patients with ME/CFS have an immunodeficiency severe enough to cause chronic enterovirus infection; although immunological abnormalities can be demonstrated, these are most likely to be consequent to infection rather than the cause of infection. However, the possible identification of virus-like particles consistent with enteroviruses in cases of encephalitis lethargica means that enteroviruses cannot be dismissed as a potential cause of at least some cases of ME/CFS and the question is being revisited with more accurate diagnostic tests. The demonstration that patients with Long Covid may have evidence of persistent viral infection in cerebrospinal fluid (CSF) and brain tissue long after the acute illness, means that there is a need to re-evaluate ME/CFS patients for the presence of persistent active viral infection.

The long history of chronic fatigue syndrome suggests that it is highly unlikely that there is a single infectious cause of ME/CFS and that multiple pathogens may be triggers. My own practice has confirmed that typical ME/CFS can be seen after a whole range of confirmed bacterial, viral, fungal, and tropical infections. In approximately half of the patients seen with ME/CFS, there is no clear antecedent infection. This means that studies aimed at identifying one single infection as the cause of all cases of chronic fatigue are likely doomed to failure.

The lack of any clear infectious or biological cause for ME/CFS and the lack of any reliable diagnostic biomarkers accentuated the trend to characterize the illness in the 1980s and 1990s and even into the 2000s as a purely psychological or somatization disorder. Derogatory terms such as 'Yuppy flu' were used and became popular for a while in the media. This stereotyping was also incorrect, as the accumulating evidence suggests that ME/CFS can affect people of any age, sex, social class, and race. What differs between these disparate groups is how, when, or even if, they present for medical care and how healthcare providers respond. In particular, in the UK, there are disproportionately fewer patients of Asian or other ethnic backgrounds presenting with ME/CFS, which is likely to be due to reduced awareness of the illness and poor access to healthcare.

A gradual change in official attitude did develop, starting with the 1996 Report commissioned by Kenneth Calman, then Chief Medical Officer in the UK, from the Royal Colleges of Physicians, General Practitioners, and Psychiatrists. The report legitimized the diagnosis and began the process of moving away from a psychological cause to a more medical basis. Kenneth Calman's successor, Liam Donaldson, commissioned a working group in 2002, which led in 2005–06 to the establishment of Department of Health-funded services in England, although none were established in Scotland or Northern Ireland. No clear model was proposed, and services developed very differently around England. In the absence of any curative treatments, the process involved confirmation of diagnosis followed by physical and psychological rehabilitation. Eventually, the responsibility for funding was developed to local commissioning organizations, supposedly ring-fenced, but financial pressures meant that many services were pared to the minimum or closed altogether. Some services were simply merged into services for patients with 'medically unexplained illness', a very inappropriate setting. Expertise that had been built up over a period of years was then diluted or lost.

In 2007 the National Institute for Clinical Excellence (NICE) in England published guidelines on CFS/ME regarding diagnosis and treatment, with treatment largely focused on a biopsychosocial model.[2] This approach was controversial at the time, and some of the authors of the report even received death threats. Despite the focus on the psychological model of treatment, the existence of NICE Guidelines required doctors and managers to recognize the illness and make some provision. In 2017, NICE declined to review the guidelines, despite significant development in the understanding of the condition but after pressure from patients and doctors reversed the decision. One of the key changes was removal of the requirement to consider graded exercise therapy and the substitution of pacing. Despite the changes and a very difficult and controversial process, new guidelines were issued in late 2021.[3]

In the USA, an influential report was produced by the Institute of Medicine in 2015.[4] This confirmed that CFS/ME was a medical not psychiatric or psychological illness. A new name was suggested in place of ME/CFS: systemic exertion intolerance disease (SEID), although there is no evidence that uptake of this new name has been widespread. UK and European guidelines continue to use the term ME/CFS.

[2] See CGC53—https://huisartsvink.files.wordpress.com/2022/02/nice-2007-me-cfs-guideline.pdf
[3] NICE Guidelines, https://www.nice.org.uk/guidance/ng206
[4] Institute of Medicine (2015), https://nap.nationalacademies.org/read/19012/chapter/1

The Medical Research Council in the UK did, after a lot of prodding, take specific steps to encourage high-quality research in the field of ME/CFS, led by Professor Stephen Holgate, having previously studiously ignored ME/CFS research proposals. The biggest driver to research came as a result of the SARS-CoV2 epidemic and the consequent appearance of Long Covid. In the UK, there is a professional association for clinical staff involved in the care of patients with ME/CFS (British Association of Clinicians in ME, BACME: *https://bacme.info* which requires paid membership). There is a European network for clinicians and researchers (EuroMENE: *https://euromene.eu/index.html*). For Long Covid, a professional organization has been set up between the NHS and the British Society for Physical and Rehabilitation Medicine (Clinical Post Covid Society *https://www.clinicalpcs.org.uk*).

The fact that significant numbers of healthcare staff developed what has been called Long Covid led to pressure to provide additional care. Regardless of the expertise developed in managing ME/CFS over the previous 12 years, services were set up from scratch, bypassing existing pathways for chronic fatigue and duplicating effort. This separation of Long Covid from ME/CFS led to a lot of ill-feeling from ME/CFS patients who viewed Long Covid patients as getting preferential treatment, when to all intents and purposes the two conditions are identical. The convergence of science confirms that the underlying pathology is similar if not identical and that the management of the two conditions should be the same and now services are beginning to join up, so that Long Covid patients can benefit from the expertise built up by the ME/CFS services. More and more research is being done comparing all aspects of ME/CFS with Long Covid and the similarities are striking (see Annesley at al 2024).

The UK Government is beginning to realize that a step change in care is required. In their interim delivery plan, published in 2024 it acknowledges that a conservative estimate of the cost to the UK of ME/CFS is around £3.3 billion based on a 0.4% prevalence (figures from 2014 to 2015).[5] 10 years on, one suspects that the true cost is much higher and then there is the cost of managing Long Covid on top of that. A study by Cambridge Econometrics estimates that the cost of Long Covid is around £1.9 billion, but if cases continue to rise, the total by 2030 might be as much as £9.3 billion.[6] These are enormous sums and concerted action to reduce the health burden will improve lives and save money in the short and medium term. Against this, the Government has invested only £314 million in providing services for Long Covid. A study from the University of Birmingham has identified additional costs in primary care for Long Covid of

---

[5] UK Government consultation outcome, *My full reality: the interim delivery plan on ME/CFS* (2024), *https://www.gov.uk/government/consultations/improving-the-experiences-of-people-with-mecfs-interim-delivery-plan/my-full-reality-the-interim-delivery-plan-on-mecfs#:~:text=The%20Living%20with%20ME%2FCFS,care%20services%2C%20welfare%20support%20and*

[6] Cambridge Econometrics (March 2024), *https://www.camecon.com/wp-content/uploads/2024/03/The-Economic-Burden-of-Long-Covid_Cambridge-Econometrics_March2024_Report-Summary.pdf*

between £23–60 million (Tufts et al., 2023), at a time when primary care is already struggling.

FURTHER READING

Annesley SJ, Missailidis D, Heng B, Josev EK, Armstrong CW. Unravelling shared mechanisms: insights from recent ME/CFS research to illuminate long COVID pathologies. *Trends Mol Med.* 2024;30:443–8. *https://doi.org/10.1016/j.mol med.2024.02.003.*

Briggs NC, Levine PH. A comparative review of systemic and neurological symptomatology in 12 outbreaks collectively described as chronic fatigue syndrome, epidemic neuromyasthenia, and myalgic encephalomyelitis. *Clin Infect Dis.* 1994;18(Supplement_1):S32–42. *https://doi.org/10.1093/clinids/18.Supplement_1.S32.*

CFS/ME Working Group. *A report of the CFS/ME working group: report to the chief medical officer of an independent working group.* Department of Health; 2002.

Dourmashkin RR, Dunn G, Castano V, McCall SA. Evidence for an enterovirus as the cause of encephalitis lethargica. *BMC Infect Dis.* 2012;12:1–21. *http://www.biomedcent ral.com/1471-2334/12/136.*

McEvedy CP, Beard AW. Royal Free epidemic of 1955: a reconsideration. *Br Med J.* 1970;1(5687):7–11. *https://doi.org/10.1136/bmj.1.5687.7.*

O'Neal AJ, Hanson MR. The enterovirus theory of disease etiology in myalgic encephalomyelitis/chronic fatigue syndrome: a critical review. *Front Med.* 2021;8:688486. *https://doi.org/10.3389/fmed.2021.688486.*

Royal Colleges of Physicians, Psychiatrists and General Practitioners. *Chronic fatigue syndrome: report of a joint working group of the Royal Colleges of Physicians, Psychiatrists and General Practitioners.* Royal College of Physicians of London; 1996.

The Medical Staff of The Royal Free Hospital. An outbreak of encephalomyelitis in the Royal Free Hospital Group, London, in 1955. *Br Med J.* 1957;2(5050):895–904.

Tufts J, Guan N, Zemedikun DT, et al. The cost of primary care consultations associated with long COVID in non-hospitalised adults: a retrospective cohort study using UK primary care data. *BMC Prim Care.* 2023;24:245. *https://doi.org/10.1186/s12 875-023-02196-1.*

Underhill R, Baillod R. Myalgic encephalomyelitis/chronic fatigue syndrome: organic disease or psychosomatic illness? A re-examination of the Royal Free Epidemic of 1955. *Medicina (Kaunas).* 2020;57(1):12. *https://doi.org/10.3390/medicina57010012.*

CHAPTER 2

When to suspect ME/CFS or Long Covid

KEY POINTS

* 'Tiredness' is a very common presentation in primary care (20% of patients).
* Fatigue and tiredness are not the same: it is crucial to distinguish between the two.
* Careful history taking is the key.
* The symptoms of chronic fatigue (including ME/CFS and Long Covid) are different from tiredness.
* Sleep is disturbed and unrefreshing in chronic fatigue.
* Post-exertional malaise is a key feature of chronic fatigue.
* Anyone of any age, sex, or race can get chronic fatigue.

2.1 What is fatigue?

Fatigue and tiredness are inevitably and frequently confused, even in the minds of healthcare workers. They are not the same. Tiredness is what you expect if you have worked or exercised hard, missed your sleep, and it is relieved by sleeping. Fatigue is not relieved by rest or sleep and is persistent. Fatigue is not unique to ME/CFS but is a consequence of many acute and chronic illnesses, many of which are discussed in later chapters. ME/CFS is the diagnosis that should be considered when other confounding medical illnesses have been excluded and nationally accepted clinical symptoms and illness duration are met.

About 20% of GP consultations are about tiredness or fatigue (known as TATT = tired all the time). In the vast majority of cases, no significant illness is underlying the presentation. Lifestyle may be a considerable contributor: over-work, juggling job and family, life stressors, etc. Two questions can separate tiredness from fatigue: i) is normal sleep refreshing? Yes = tired, No = fatigued; ii) Does activity make the person sleep better? Yes = tired, No = fatigued. This is a very important sieve. People who fall into the fatigue group by this test may still have medical problems, not necessarily ME/CFS. People who fall into the tired group may still have medical problems, or maybe working too hard, exercising too hard, or be sleep deprived. This highlights key features of ME/CFS and Long Covid: sleep is unrefreshing, sleep disturbance is common, and fatigue is disproportionate to activity and there is post-exertional malaise. For Long Covid, clearly the onset after a confirmed (by antigen or molecular viral test) episode of infection with SARS-CoV2 is required.

For doctors in primary care, there are useful resources available to guide the diagnostic process.[1] Distinguishing between tiredness and fatigue is the crucial first step in making or refuting a diagnosis of chronic fatigue (any cause). Only once this has been done can an appropriate consideration of the differential diagnosis and relevant further investigations be undertaken. The key to correct diagnosis is invariably in the history and this means giving the patient time to tell their story.

Fatigue is common after even quite minor illnesses, like the common cold, but this will usually resolve rapidly after a few days to two weeks. Fatigue persisting beyond two weeks is abnormal. Now, with increased scrutiny, chronic fatigue is recognized even after a common cold. Fatigue is the body's normal response to infection or inflammation and is mediated by changes in the levels of cytokines. It is crucial at the first presentation to look for red flag signs indicating a serious underlying cause for fatigue. These include weight loss, lymphadenopathy, any signs suggestive of malignancy, focal neurological signs, signs and symptoms of sleep apnoea, inflammatory diseases, cardiac disease, and respiratory disease. The spectrum of the differential diagnosis is discussed in more detail in the next chapter.

Chronic fatigue syndrome should be considered only when careful consideration has excluded other serious pathology.

For those who are fit and very active, that fitness will start to disappear from two weeks onwards after an illness that causes fatigue and will continue to decline. Keeping fit is like trying to climb a greasy pole: you have to keep working to stay in the same place and work harder to climb higher. If you stop climbing, you slide back to the bottom and have to start again to regain fitness. Therefore, the impact of prolonged fatigue on a person's physiology starts very quickly. Ideally, therefore, interventions need to start early too. Telling a patient to go away and that everything will just get better is unhelpful.

FURTHER READING

Stadje R, Dornieden K, Baum E, et al. The differential diagnosis of tiredness: a systematic review. *BMC Fam Pract.* 2016;17(1):1–1. *https://doi.org/10.1186/s12875-016-0545-5.*

2.2 Other symptoms

Chronic fatigue syndrome (ME/CFS, Long Covid) is usually accompanied by a range of other symptoms. These include joint and muscle pains, headaches, word-finding difficulty, 'brain fog', sleep disturbance, dizziness, temperature

---

[1] NICE Guidelines, *https://cks.nice.org.uk/topics/tiredness-fatigue-in-adults/*

disturbance, sore throats, swollen glands, sensory intolerance (light, noise, smells, tastes), and bowel and bladder symptoms. Breathing difficulty may be present, often described as 'air hunger', which is different from shortness of breath (breathing tests tend to be normal). A boom-and-bust pattern of activity is typical, where a marginal improvement is followed by an inappropriate increase in activity which in turn leads to a flare of symptoms (post-exertional malaise). Long Covid patients may also have persistent anosmia, a very specific marker of SARS-CoV2 infection. Because SARS-CoV2 is a respiratory pathogen, patients may have actual lung damage as a consequence of the acute illness, which needs to be distinguished from the 'air hunger' which has a neurogenic basis. The key symptoms and diagnostic criteria are described in more detail in Chapter 3.

The symptoms of chronic fatigue are fairly stereotyped and the majority of the patients will have most but not necessarily all of the symptoms. Not all the symptoms will be present all the time. The key features to look out for are the neurocognitive problems: word-finding difficulty; memory problems in association with unrefreshing sleep. However, the list of other conditions that can present in a similar way is very long and a detailed review is required to exclude these (see Chapter 4.1).

For specialists seeing many patients over a long period of time, it is reassuring how consistent the symptomatology is for ME/CFS. This makes it easier to recognize deviations from the expected pattern that may suggest an alternative diagnosis and will lead to alternative lines of questioning. It is harder for non-specialists to pick out this pattern. I was taught as a medical student and trainee doctor that the history is the key to diagnosis: you should have a pretty good idea of the diagnosis by the time you have taken a history (assuming you have been thorough). Examination should serve to confirm (or occasionally refute) your preliminary diagnosis. Equally if you have no idea of a diagnosis at the end of the history and examination, it is unlikely that scattergun investigation will help either!

Taking time over the history is therefore the most important part of effective diagnosis. This can be difficult in the current state of the NHS with pressure to see ever more patients in the shortest possible time. In the absence of any simple diagnostic tests for ME/CFS, the history taking skill is therefore the most effective diagnostic tool. This should not be a rote exercise: concentration is required to pick up on subtle clues that may point to other illness. Long Covid is slightly easier to diagnose due to the link with an identifiable episode of infection which is readily confirmed with widely available tests.

One of the most striking examples of this was the case of a widowed lady in her 60s, referred with suspected chronic fatigue by her GP. She had no children and no family. The history taking was proceeding along typical ME/CFS lines, when I asked a question about any past stressors. The lady paused and didn't answer immediately and then said a tentative 'no', while her face and tone of her voice said 'yes'. There was just one moment when I could either take her answer at face value or stop and challenge her. I chose the latter and asked whether there really was anything else. She then told me the story of her life: she had been married, but her husband had died a few years ago. He was abusive to her, physically and mentally. She was more or less kept a prisoner in her own house and her husband rented her out regularly for sex to his friends. I was the first person she had dared to tell about this awful story; she had never told her GP. The more she talked, the clearer it became that she was suffering from severe post-traumatic stress disorder (PTSD), with flashbacks to the worst times of her married life, and with very disturbed sleep accompanied by nightmares. From being a 'routine' ME/CFS referral, the history had revealed something completely different. I thought afterwards how easy it would have been to miss the singular moment when the patient offered me the chance to ask more detailed questions and simply have carried on with the rest of the history. This was such an eye opener. She wanted to tell someone, but needed them to ask first. I had a very good medical student, who was interested in ME/CFS sitting in with me for this consultation and I could see the look of shock on her face as the patient explained her personal history. Afterwards, we discussed just how important it is in a history to follow up on even tiny clues and not just press on like an automaton. It also makes the point that face-to-face consultation with a human is required to pick up the discrepancy between what was said and how it was said and what the face said. A telephone consultation would have completely missed this. I doubt whether AI would have identified it either.

For Long Covid, the diagnosis is made somewhat easier by a preceding history of COVID-19. The widespread use of testing, including the ability to purchase antigen test kits over the counter, means that linking persistent fatigue to a recent episode of COVID-19 infection is much easier.

FURTHER READING

Wong TL, Weitzer DJ. Long COVID and myalgic encephalomyelitis/chronic fatigue syndrome (ME/CFS)—a systemic review and comparison of clinical presentation and symptomatology. *Medicina*. 2021;**57**(5):418. *https://doi.org/10.3390/medicina5 7050418*.

2.3 Who gets chronic fatigue?

ME/CFS is perhaps perceived as a rare disease. However, the best estimate is a predicted prevalence of 857/100,000, making it a relatively common illness. There is also a perception that it is predominantly a female illness, but the relative risk for females is similar to males, except in the under 9s, when boys predominate. However, this does depend on which studies you look at, as females may comprise up to 80% in some studies. All age groups are affected from early childhood to the very elderly, peaking in early to middle adulthood. Selection bias in studies may account for the differing sex and age ratios.

Risk factors for the development of ME/CFS identified in studies include the following:

History of frequents colds or other infections
Being Single
Lower Income
Family history of anxiety
Other family members with ME/CFS

Studies have also shown that patients presenting with ME/CFS often have a history of major stressful events in the preceding 2 years. This can be redundancy, divorce, or bereavement but can include major life stress. For example, there was a surge of cases in North Cumbria following two major flooding events. These cases were invariably people who had been flooded out of their homes or businesses and had lost possessions or sometimes their livelihoods and had to leave their homes for prolonged periods.

Severe ME/CFS is more likely in younger patients and those with a family history of neurological disease. Abuse as a child has been identified in some studies and should certainly be considered during history taking.

The genetics of ME/CFS is complex (discussed further in Chapter 5). At least 422 loci have been identified that may impact on susceptibility to ME/CFS. It is quite clear that it is not a simple genetic illness. It is likely that the genetic susceptibility will be linked specifically to the genes controlling responses to specific infections.

There is a clear perception that Black and ethnic minorities are underrepresented in studies on ME/CFS, even though there is no evidence to suggest that these groups are less likely to be affected by ME/CFS or by Long Covid. In fact, recent research on Long Covid suggests that ethnic minorities may be *more* likely to develop Long Covid (see Section 2.4). There are many potential reasons for this, including lack of access to healthcare, other social and deprivation-related issues that assume greater importance, other health issues and non-engagement with orthodox medicine. In fact, symptom scores in Black and ethnic minorities tend to be much higher. Social status has a profound impact on access to healthcare, and white middle-class patients are more likely to present and demand further investigation. The paradigm that ethnic minorities may present with more general physical symptoms or medically unexplained symptoms has however been challenged (Evangelidou et al., 2020).

In some Asian communities in the UK, communication is difficult, as some older patients do not speak English, and their access to healthcare is controlled by other family members. Often histories for female patients are initially only obtained through a (male) family member, so identifying the true basis of the symptoms can be extremely difficult unless an unrelated same-sex interpreter is used. There can be differences between the doctor and the patient in understanding the meaning of questions about symptoms. Unfortunately, many of the research studies in ME/CFS are heavily weighted towards white Caucasian patients.

FURTHER READING

Evangelidou S, NeMoyer A, Cruz-Gonzalez M, O'Malley I, Alegría M. Racial/ethnic differences in general physical symptoms and medically unexplained physical symptoms: investigating the role of education. *Cultur Divers Ethnic Minor Psychol.* 2020;26(4):557. *https://doi.org/10.1037/cdp0000319.*

Jason LA, Torres C. Differences in symptoms among Black and white patients with ME/CFS. *J Clin Med.* 2022;11:6708. *https://doi.org/10.3390/jcm11226708.*

Lacerda EM, Geraghty K, Kingdon CC, et al. A logistic regression analysis of risk factors in ME/CFS pathogenesis. *BMC Neurol.* 2019;19:275. *https://doi.org/10.1186/s12 883-019-1468-2.*

Schlauch KA, Khaiboullina SF, De Meirleir KL, et al. Genome-wide association analysis identifies genetic variations in subjects with myalgic encephalomyelitis/chronic fatigue syndrome. *Transl Psychiatry.* 2016;6(2):e730. *https://doi.org/10.1038/tp.2015.208.*

Valdez AR, Hancock EE, Adebayo S, et al. Estimating prevalence, demographics, and costs of ME/CFS using large scale medical claims data and machine learning. *Front Pediatr.* 2019;6:412. *https://doi.org/10.3389/fped.2018.00412.*

2.4 Who gets Long Covid?

Studies have shown that the risk of developing Long Covid is greater in those with severe acute disease, those with tachycardia, which may indicate underlying myocarditis, and those with antibiotics use (a surrogate marker of severity). However, Long Covid may be seen after mild infection. While female sex has been suggested as a risk factor, multivariate analysis has refuted this. Older age at infection is a risk factor. Blood group B appears to be protective. The highest incidence appears to have occurred with the original variants of SARS-CoV2, with later strains being less likely to cause it. Being unvaccinated is a risk factor and evidence to support the hypothesis that vaccination triggers Long Covid is very weak. The consensus is that vaccination is likely to be protective. A very recent study (Wang et al., 2024) of over 1.5 million adults with COVID-19 in the UK has suggested that risk factors for Long Covid included being female, non-white, obese and having pre-existing medical or mental health conditions (anxiety/depression, type 2 diabetes, and somatic symptom disorders).

The most recent large study (Yan Tie et al., 2024) found that Long Covid developed in 10.4% of unvaccinated people infected with the original strain, 9.5% infected with the Delta strain and 7.5% with the Omicron strain. Of those who had been vaccinated, Long Covid occurred in 5.3% infected with the original stain and 3.5% of those infected with Omicron. It was also clear that the individual strains had distinctive patterns of which organs were affected. Later strains have seemed to cause more metabolic and gastrointestinal symptoms.

After SARS-CoV2, 7.5% of people will still be symptomatic 12 weeks after acute infection and 5.2% after a year, but for unvaccinated 17.2% still had symptoms after 2 years. It also appears that those with asthma and rheumatoid arthritis may be more likely to develop it. Variations in the gene FOXP4, which is involved in lung function, are associated with the severity of COVID-19 infection and therefore may increase the risk of developing Long Covid.

A large Danish study has suggested that ethnic minorities may be more likely to develop Long Covid compared to ethnic Danes and, in particular, to have more cardiopulmonary symptoms as a result (Mkoma et al., 2024). Similar results have been obtained in the USA (Khullar et al., 2023).

FURTHER READING

Guzman-Esquivel J, Mendoza-Hernandez MA, Guzman-Solorzano HP, et al. Clinical characteristics in the acute phase of COVID-19 that predict long COVID: tachycardia, myalgias, severity, and use of antibiotics as main risk factors, while education and blood group B are protective. *Healthcare*. 2023;11(2):197. *https://doi.org/10.3390/healthcare1 1020197.*

Khullar D, Zhang Y, Zang C, et al. Racial/ethnic disparities in post-acute sequelae of SARS-CoV-2 infection in New York: an EHR-based cohort study from the RECOVER program. *J Gen Int Med*. 2023;38(5):1127–36. *https://doi.org/10.1007/s11 606-022-07997-1.*

Luo YS, Zhang K, Cheng ZS. Absence of association between a long COVID and severe COVID-19 risk variant of FOXP4 and lung cancer. *Front Genet*. 2023;14:1258829. *https://doi.org/10.3389/fgene.2023.1258829.*

Mkoma GF, Agyemang C, Benfield T, et al. Risk of long COVID and associated symptoms after acute SARS-COV-2 infection in ethnic minorities: A nationwide register-linked cohort study in Denmark. *PLoS Med*. 2024;21(2):e1004280. *https://doi.org/10.1371/ journal.pmed.1004280.*

Wang HI, Doran T, Crooks MG, et al. Prevalence, risk factors and characterisation of individuals with long COVID using electronic health records in over 1.5 million COVID cases in England. *J Infect*. 2024;89:106235. *https://doi.org/10.1016/j.jinf.2024.106235.*

Xie Y, Choi T, Al-Aly Z. Postacute sequelae of SARS-CoV-2 infection in the pre-Delta, Delta, and Omicron eras. *N Engl J Med*. 2024;391(6):515–25. *https://doi.org/10.1056/ NEJMoa2403211.*

The diagnosis of ME/CFS and Long Covid

3.1 Diagnosis and diagnostic tests

Several diagnoses and diagnostic criteria have been used over the years (Oxford, CDC/Fukuda, Canadian, NICE, dePaul), but none are perfect. Even attempts to generate international consensus have been difficult. More recent criteria have been published by the Institute of Medicine (IoM) in the USA in 2015 and by the European ME Network in 2021. The latter discusses previous diagnostic criteria and criteria for children (also covered in the IoM document). Mostly they are used for classification for research purposes and their clinical utility is variable. None of these criteria reliably distinguish by themselves between primary and secondary fatigue.

The CDC website has a summary of the IoM (2015) criteria, which are included in Box 3.1.

The NICE guidelines (2021) have simpler criteria: see Box 3.2.

However, even now there are ongoing discussion about the appropriateness of the guidelines, with attempts to refine the accuracy (see Conroy et al 2023) and this process is likely to continue as the science changes our views and new diagnostic tests become available.

Patients may well have used other resources such as the internet to research their own symptoms. This makes obtaining an uncontaminated history difficult, and patients will often present their symptoms in a way that they believe confirms their theory that they have ME/CFS. They frequently attend with folders of information, including scientific papers. This may require the clinician to make use of directed questioning about specific symptoms, even though we are taught

Box 3.1 Institute of Medicine Criteria for ME/CFS 2015

The 2015 IoM diagnostic criteria for ME/CFS in adults and children state that **three symptoms and at least one of two additional manifestations are required** for diagnosis. The three required symptoms are:

1. **A substantial reduction or impairment in the ability to engage in pre-illness levels of activity** (occupational, educational, social, or personal life) that:
   1. lasts for more than 6 months
   2. is accompanied by fatigue that is:
      1. often profound
      2. of new onset (not life-long)
      3. not the result of ongoing or unusual excessive exertion
      4. not substantially alleviated by rest
2. **Post-exertional malaise (PEM)***—worsening of symptoms after physical, mental, or emotional exertion that would not have caused a problem before the illness. PEM often puts the patient in relapse that may last days, weeks, or even longer. For some patients, sensory overload (light and sound) can induce PEM. The symptoms typically get worse 12 to 48 hours after the activity or exposure and can last for days or even weeks.
3. **Unrefreshing sleep***—patients with ME/CFS may not feel better or less tired even after a full night of sleep despite the absence of specific objective sleep alterations.

At least one of the following **two additional manifestations** must be present:

1. **Cognitive impairment***—patients have problems with thinking, memory, executive function, and information processing, as well as attention deficit and impaired psychomotor functions. All can be exacerbated by exertion, effort, prolonged upright posture, stress, or time pressure, and may have serious consequences on a patient's ability to maintain a job or attend school full time.
2. **Orthostatic intolerance**—patients develop a worsening of symptoms upon assuming and maintaining an upright posture as measured by objective heart rate and blood pressure abnormalities during standing, bedside orthostatic vital signs, or head-up tilt testing. Orthostatic symptoms, including lightheadedness, fainting, increased fatigue, cognitive worsening, headaches, or nausea, are worsened with quiet upright posture (either standing or sitting) during day-to-day life and are improved

continued >

Box 3.1 (Continued)

(though not necessarily fully resolved) with lying down. Orthostatic intolerance is often the most bothersome manifestation of ME/CFS among adolescents.

*The frequency and severity of these symptoms need to be evaluated. The IoM committee specified that **'The diagnosis of ME/CFS should be questioned if patients do not have these symptoms at least half of the time with moderate, substantial, or severe intensity'.**

Other common symptoms of ME/CFS

Many people with ME/CFS also have other symptoms. Additional common symptoms include:

• Muscle pain
• Pain in the joints without swelling or redness
• Headaches of a new type, pattern, or severity
• Swollen or tender lymph nodes in the neck or armpit
• A sore throat that is frequent or recurring
• Chills and night sweats
• Visual disturbances
• Sensitivity to light and sound
• Nausea
• Allergies or sensitivities to foods, odours, chemicals, or medications

Source: data from IoM 2015 Diagnostic Criteria | ME/CFS | CDC; see: *https://nap.nationalacademies. org/resource/19012/MECFScliniciansguide.pdf.*

---

to use open questions wherever possible. Very rarely it is necessary to use questions where the answer should be a negative, to see whether the patient is simply saying they have any symptoms that the doctor mentions: I use the 'do you have green urine' question. This usually works, although I did have one patient who actually did have confirmed green urine (the laboratory identified methylene blue in the urine, which we discovered came from a curious over-the-counter (OTC) liver 'tonic' that the patient was using, even in hospital)! So even the whackiest questions sometimes still give justified positive answers!

Two types of ME/CFS are identifiable, those with a definable starting point for their symptoms, usually following symptoms compatible with an acute infection, and a group with a gradual onset and no obvious pointers to a triggering event. It is unclear at present whether these groups are physiologically distinct, but their symptomatology is identical, and so it seems are their outcomes.

In terms of clinical history, a more detailed list of symptoms should be explored, with the view of picking up pointers to other fatigue-inducing conditions or red-flag symptoms (see next section).

> **Box 3.2** Diagnostic criteria ME/CFS—NICE guidelines 2021
>
> All of these symptoms should be present:
>
> - Debilitating fatigue that is worsened by activity, is not caused by excessive cognitive, physical, emotional, or social exertion, and is not significantly relieved by rest.
> - Post-exertional malaise after activity in which the worsening of symptoms:
>   - o is often delayed in onset by hours or days
>   - o is disproportionate to the activity
>   - o has a prolonged recovery time that may last hours, days, weeks, or longer.
> - Unrefreshing sleep or sleep disturbance (or both), which may include:
>   - o feeling exhausted, feeling flu-like, and stiff on waking
>   - o broken or shallow sleep, altered sleep pattern, or hypersomnia.
> - Cognitive difficulties (sometimes described as 'brain fog'), which may include problems finding words or numbers, difficulty in speaking, slowed responsiveness, short-term memory problems, and difficulty concentrating or multitasking.
>
> Suspect ME/CFS if:
>
> - the person has had all of the persistent symptoms in Box 3.2 for a minimum of 6 weeks in adults and 4 weeks in children and young people, **and**
> - the person's ability to engage in occupational, educational, social or personal activities is significantly reduced from pre-illness levels, **and**
> - symptoms are not explained by another condition.
>
> The important feature of these revised guidelines is that the time frame for making the diagnosis has been shortened considerably, from 4 months in the first iteration of the Guidelines (CGC53) to 6 weeks for adults.
>

Specific diagnostic criteria have been established for Long Covid (Shah et al., 2021).[1] Key features are summarized in Box 3.3. There must be evidence of SARS-CoV2 infection.

As will be immediately apparent, the list of symptoms accurately matches this of ME/CFS, with the exception of disordered taste and smell. However, disturbed taste and abnormal perceptions of smells also occur in ME/CFS, as part of sensory intolerance. Complete anosmia however does not seem to occur in ME/

---

[1] NICE, *COVID-19 rapid guideline: managing the long-term effects of COVID-19* (2020, updated 2024) *www.nice.org.uk/guidance/ng188*

Box 3.3 Diagnostic features of Long Covid

Respiratory symptoms: breathlessness, cough
Cardiovascular symptoms: chest tightness, chest pain, palpitations
Generalized symptoms: fatigue, fever, pain
Neurological symptoms: cognitive impairment (brain fog, loss of concentration or memory issues), headache, sleep disturbance, peripheral neuropathy symptoms (pins and needles, numbness), dizziness, delirium (in older populations).
Gastrointestinal symptoms: abdominal pain, nausea, diarrhoea, anorexia, and reduced appetite (older populations)
Musculoskeletal symptoms: joint pain, muscle pain
Psychological/psychiatric symptoms: symptoms of depression, symptoms of anxiety
Ear, nose and throat symptoms: tinnitus, earache, sore throat, loss of taste, and/or smell
Dermatological: skin rashes

CFS. Even allowing for the clear association with SARS-CoV2 infection, a recent study has found that <1% of patients with symptoms compatible with Long Covid at 12 weeks after infection were actually diagnosed with Long Covid!

FURTHER READING

Brown AA, Jason LA, Evans MA, Flores S. Contrasting case definitions: the ME International Consensus Criteria vs. the Fukuda et al. CFS criteria. *N Am J Psychol.* 2013;15(1):103.

Carruthers BM, Jain AK, De Meirleir KL, et al. Myalgic encephalomyelitis/chronic fatigue syndrome: clinical working case definition, diagnostic and treatment protocols. *J Chronic Fatigue Syndr.* 2003;11(1):7–115.

Committee on the Diagnostic Criteria for Myalgic Encephalomyelitis/Chronic Fatigue Syndrome; Board on the Health of Select Populations; Institute of Medicine. *Beyond myalgic encephalomyelitis/chronic fatigue syndrome: redefining an illness.* National Academies Press (US); 2015.

Conroy KE, Islam MF, Jason LA. Evaluating case diagnostic criteria for myalgic encephalomyelitis/chronic fatigue syndrome (ME/CFS): toward an empirical case definition. *Disabil Rehabil.* 2023;45(5):840–7. *https://doi.org/10.1080/09638 288.2022.2043462.*

Fukuda K, Straus SE, Hickie I, Sharpe MC, Dobbins JG, Komaroff A, International Chronic Fatigue Syndrome Study Group. The chronic fatigue syndrome: a comprehensive approach to its definition and study. *Ann Int Med.* 1994;121(12):953–9. *https://doi.org/10.7326/0003-4819-121-12-199412150-00009.*

Kingdon C, Lowe A, Shepherd C, Nacul L. What primary care practitioners need to know about the new NICE guideline for myalgic encephalomyelitis/chronic fatigue syndrome in adults. *InHealthcare.* 2022;10(12):2438. *https://doi.org/10.3390/healthcare10122438.*

Nacul L, Authier FJ, Scheibenbogen C, et al. European Network on Myalgic Encephalomyelitis/Chronic Fatigue Syndrome (EUROMENE): expert consensus on the diagnosis, service provision, and care of people with ME/CFS in Europe. *Medicina.* 2021;57(5):510. *https://doi.org/10.3390/medicina57050510.*

Nurek M, Rayner C, Freyer A, Taylor S, Järte L, MacDermott N, Delaney BC. Recommendations for the recognition, diagnosis, and management of long COVID: a Delphi study. *Br J Gen Pract.* 2021; 71 (712):e815–25. *https://doi.org/10.3399/BJGP.2021.0265.*

Shah W, Hillman T, Playford ED, Hishmeh L. Managing the long term effects of COVID-19: summary of NICE, SIGN, and RCGP rapid guideline. *BMJ.* 2021;372. *http://dx.doi.org/10.1136/bmj.n136.*

Sisó-Almirall A, Brito-Zerón P, Conangla Ferrin L, et al. Long COVID-19: proposed primary care clinical guidelines for diagnosis and disease management. *Int J Environ Res Public Health.* 2021;18(8):4350. *https://doi.org/10.3390/ijerph18084350.*

Twisk F. Myalgic encephalomyelitis or what? The International Consensus Criteria. *Diagnostics.* 2018;9(1):1. *htttps://doi.org/10.3390/diagnostics9010001.*

Yelin D, Moschopoulos CD, Margalit I, et al. ESCMID rapid guidelines for assessment and management of long COVID. *Clin Microbiol Infect.* 2022;28(7):955–72. *https://doi.org/10.1016/j.cmi.2022.02.018.*

3.2 History and examination

Until such time as we have robust biomarkers for the diagnosis of ME/CFS and Long Covid, the diagnosis is dependent on accurate history taking, followed by examination. The findings then need to be matched against the established criteria. It is crucial that practitioners are alert to the possibilities of other causes of chronic fatigue (see Chapter 4.1). For Long Covid, the diagnostic process is somewhat simplified by the presence of robust evidence of prior infection with SARS-CoV2, but it remains important to ensure that any other potential alternative causes for chronic fatigue are still excluded.

3.2.1 The history

Key areas to explore in the history:

1. Prolonged debilitating fatigue (not tiredness) made worse by activity. This should be of at least 6 weeks duration in adults and less in children. The fatigue should have an impact on functional capacity and it is helpful to ascertain the patient's pre-morbid functional capacity to get an idea of

their baseline capability. This will impact how they perceive fatigue. A super-fit ultra-marathon runner will notice fatigue at a higher level of activity but feel more disabled by it than someone who is relatively inactive. For a diagnosis of Long Covid, exploration of the history for evidence of SARS-CoV2 infection is essential and should include timing, severity, need for hospitalization, and acute complications, which have a bearing on the likelihood of developing Long Covid. Vaccination status should be checked.

2. Generalized muscular and joint pains without evidence of joint swelling, made worse by exercise. Identify how much physical activity is required. The post-exertional fatigue (malaise) after exercise may not be immediate and may be 24-48 hours later. Symptoms overlap considerably with fibromyalgia.

3. Neurocognitive impairment ('brain fog')—reduced short-term memory and concentration (obtain specific examples, for example ability to read and follow a plot or watch a film). Long-term memory is usually intact.

4. Word-finding difficulty. This may be apparent during the history but check for examples.

5. Disturbance of sleep and/or feeling unrefreshed by sleep. Typically, there is difficulty in getting off to sleep, and sleep is restless. On waking fatigue is present, unlike tiredness, when sleep will refresh.

6. Headache—usually generalized. Distinguish focal headache and migraine. Check for scalp tenderness (giant cell arteritis?) and visual disturbance (migraine, giant cell arteritis).

7. Dizziness (non-rotational); shakiness (not tremor). Dizziness may be due to postural hypotension or tachycardia, so this should be followed up on examination.

8. Increased frequency of sore throats and swollen glands. The swelling tends to be small and quite tender. Examination should look for evidence of large, non-tender nodes, which may be a marker of lymphoma.

9. Temperature disturbance. This is usually environmentally inappropriate temperature, for example, being hot when others are cold and vice versa.

10. Sensory intolerance is common. This includes sensitivity to loud noises, bright lights, strong smells, and strong tastes. There may be hyperalgesia, where light touch is perceived as painful. Severe sensory intolerance is a feature seen in severe ME/CFS. It can cause difficulties in managing patients in standard healthcare environments.

11. Evidence of 'boom and bust' cycles of activity followed by inactivity due to worsening symptoms.

12. Irritable bowel symptoms (IBS: nausea, bloating, abdominal discomfort/cramps, diarrhoea or constipation, or alternating bowel habits). Almost

all patients with ME/CFS have IBS. If IBS symptoms are absent, then look harder for other explanations for the fatigue.

13. Irritable bladder symptoms. These can include dysuria, and bladder pain.

14. Autonomic features: pre-syncope, syncope, positional tachycardia, abnormal sweating. Autonomic abnormalities may be present even if there is no history of dizziness or faintness. Autonomic features are likely to be most marked in patients with severe disease and those who are bed bound. Lack of time spent in the vertical position leads to atrophy of the autonomic reflexes that maintain blood pressure in the vertical position under gravity, although there is a primary autonomic failure in ME/CFS as well.

15. Breathing problems, usually described as 'air hunger' rather than shortness of breath. Asthma and chronic obstructive pulmonary disorder (COPD) may need to be excluded. In suspected Long Covid post-infectious lung damage (from infection directly or as a result of pulmonary emboli) need to be excluded.

16. Other features that are strongly associated with chronic fatigue syndrome include atypical facial pain and temporomandibular joint disorder.

17. Psychosocial stressors are usually increased in the period preceding the onset of fatigue (bereavement, divorce, redundancy, etc.) and should be noted. Abnormal bereavement reactions and post-traumatic stress disorder should be identified and referred for counselling through other channels, if this is identified as the major source of symptoms.

18. Check to see whether there is any family history of similar illnesses.

19. The patient's list of medications should be carefully checked for drugs that may cause fatigue. For example, pain treated with minor (or even major) opiates which will contribute to fatigue.

It is important during the history to identify non-CFS features, in particular:

1. Evidence of a primary sleep disorder (excessive or inappropriate somnolence, cataplexy; sleep reversal): a sleep diary may be helpful in elucidating these. Consider rapid eye movement (REM) sleep disorder in older patients: disturbed sleep with acting out of violent dreams is typical. Circadian rhythm disorder in younger patients is characterized by sleep reversal, being awake at night, and asleep in the day. Shift-workers can develop very marked sleep disturbance and chronic fatigue over time.

2. Evidence for sleep apnoea. The history from a partner is most valuable here, with loud snoring and witnessed apnoeic spells. Examination is valuable to identify the typical neck and pharyngeal shape. The Epworth sleep score (ESS) for sleep apnoea may help but is not specific. A low ESS but with a typical neck shape and confirmed history of snoring may still merit investigation for sleep apnoea.

3. Evidence for a primary psychiatric disorder: depression, bipolar disorder, severe anxiety, OCD, psychosis (as secondary depression and anxiety can accompany ME/CFS this can be difficult—if there is doubt discuss with psychologist/psychiatrist). Also consider the possibility of an autistic spectrum disorder.

4. Evidence for a primary neurological disorder. On the history, check for localized transient or persistent weakness, tremor, gait abnormalities, and double vision. Unilateral neurological symptoms indicate a possible alternative diagnosis. Any suggestion of any of these should prompt a full neurological examination and possibly a formal neurological opinion.

5. Evidence for arthritis (swollen tender joints with restricted movement) or significant joint hypermobility.

7. Evidence for documented organ-based disease (chronic lung, cardiac, liver, renal, and musculoskeletal disorders)

8. Evidence of endocrine disorder (changes in menstruation, libido, alopecia, unexpected weight gain/loss in thyroid disease).

9. Evidence for malignant disease. Fatigue may be an early feature of malignancy and can also herald relapse in those with previously treated cancer. Sudden weight loss and loss of appetite are highly suspicious. A thorough systems enquiry may identify other unsuspected pointers.

These are discussed in the next chapter under secondary causes of fatigue.

The history also needs to address family and social circumstances, past medical history, and medication. It is important to ask specifically about past stressors, and consider checking for past abuse (physical, sexual, mental) and the use of illicit drugs, as well as alcohol.

3.2.2 Examination

Most of the diagnosis is based on the history. However, a thorough physical examination is mandatory, checking skin, heart, lungs, abdomen, musculoskeletal, and neurological systems. Consider in older patients whether there is a need for dementia screening.

1. Check for clinical signs associated with sleep apnoea, such as neck size and shape and pharyngeal appearance (Use the Mallampatti scoring system for pharyngeal appearance).

2. In the neurological examination, check for muscle tenderness and wasting, fasciculation, tremor, gait and balance, focal muscle power, reflexes, sensation, cerebellar signs, vision, fundoscopy. In particular, look for unilateral neurological signs (unlikely in ME/CFS).

3. In the musculoskeletal system, check for hypermobility and skin elasticity. Look for joint swelling and inflammation and check range of movement. Check for point tenderness that may indicate fibromyalgia.

4. Check for physical signs of thyroid disease: exophthalmos, lid lag, resting tachycardia, weight loss or gain, myxoedema, signs of Addison's disease (palmar pigmentation).

5. Check lymph nodes for size and shape and check size of spleen.

6. Check for postural hypotension and/or tachycardia.

7. Any checks for malignant disease if there are any suspicious features in the history (e.g. rectal examination, examination of breasts).

3.2.3 Diagnostic formulation

At the end of the history and examination, the practitioner should have a very good idea of the diagnosis, at least to the extent of understanding whether ME/CFS or Long Covid is likely or whether an alternative fatiguing condition is the cause of symptoms. If there are unusual symptoms and/or signs, then further investigation over and above the recommended baseline tests may be appropriate. Embarking on rafts of tests, where there are no real pointers justifying them, is wasteful and can be confusing, as the more tests that are carried out, the more likely that an abnormal result is identified that has nothing to do with the reason that the patient presented. This may lead to wild goose chases, which in turn can lead to a complete loss of focus on why the patient originally presented.

Where the diagnosis is fairly clear, further investigation beyond the baseline (see next section) is unhelpful and prolongs the uncertainty for the patient, possibly raising false hopes. Particularly in hospital there is often a presumption on the part of the patient/patient's relatives that further investigations will be required, and this needs to be headed off at the outset, when there is no clinical justification. The degree of certainty for the doctor will depend on the thoroughness of the history and examination and the doctor's experience.

They doctor will need to summarize their conclusions for the patient. This needs to be in clear terms and be followed by a discussion of what the diagnosis means and what the next steps should be. This will vary according to whether the patient's illness is of recent onset or longer standing.

3.2.4 Diagnosis in children

While this is a book about the diagnosis in adults (over 16), the NICE guidelines also address the diagnosis in children. It has always been agreed that children with persistent fatigue should be investigated and referred early to paediatric services. The list of alternative potential diagnoses will be different from adults, and includes acute haematological malignancies and other tumours, other organ-based diseases (glomerulonephritis, cystic fibrosis), childhood arthritis (Still's disease, juvenile rheumatoid arthritis, polymyositis, vasculitis) and diseases that can present at any age such as coeliac disease and inflammatory bowel disease. School refusal, pervasive refusal, and eating disorders may also be accompanied or present with fatigue. Factitious illness and Münchausen syndrome by proxy also need to be considered. Consideration should always be given to the possibilities of bullying and child abuse.

FURTHER READING

Nacul L, Authier FJ, Scheibenbogen C, et al. European Network on Myalgic Encephalomyelitis/Chronic Fatigue Syndrome (EUROMENE): expert consensus on the diagnosis, service provision, and care of people with ME/CFS in Europe. *Medicina*. 2021;**57**(5):510. *https://doi.org/10.3390/medicina57050510*.

National Institute for Health and Care Excellence, Royal College of General Practitioners, Healthcare Improvement Scotland SIGN. *COVID-19 rapid guideline: managing the long-term effects of COVID-19*. 2020. *https://www.nice.org.uk/guidance/ng188*.

NICE Guideline NG206. Myalgic encephalomyelitis/chronic fatigue syndrome: diagnosis and management. 2021. *https://www.nice.org.uk/guidance/ng206*.

Rowe PC, Underhill RA, Friedman KJ, et al. Myalgic encephalomyelitis/chronic fatigue syndrome diagnosis and management in young people: a primer. Front Pediatr. 2017;**5**:121. *https://doi.org/10.3389/fped.2017.00121*.

Shah W, Hillman T, Playford ED, Hishmeh L. Managing the long term effects of covid-19: summary of NICE, SIGN, and RCGP rapid guideline. *BMJ*. 2021;**372**. *http://dx.doi.org/10.1136/bmj.n136*.

3.3 Investigations

A basic screen of blood tests is recommended for all patients presenting with prolonged fatigue for the first time and where there are no other obvious medical causes. These have been listed in the NICE guidelines cited in the previous section.

These should include:

Full blood count: this gives information on whether anaemia is present and also the type of anaemia (due to deficiency of vitamins B_{12} or folic acid, or of iron). It also provides information on the white blood cells.

Inflammatory markers: erythrocyte sedimentation rate (ESR) AND C-reactive protein. Both are required as they give *different* information about the type of inflammation present. The analogy is with diabetes: glucose levels tell you the state of the blood sugar now, while glycated haemoglobin tells what the blood sugar has been over the last few weeks. C-reactive protein (CRP) measures inflammation in the past few hours but the ESR tells about inflammation over the last three weeks. Some laboratories inappropriately try and offer only one. If either or both are raised, symptoms are unlikely to be caused by ME/CFS or Long Covid.

Creatinine and electrolytes, with eGFR: creatinine is a breakdown product of protein that is excreted by the kidneys. A raised or rising level suggests that the kidneys are not working. The eGFR (estimated glomerular filtration rate) is a calculation based on the creatine which estimates the degree of kidney function.

Glucose and/or HbA1c
Liver function tests
Thyroid function tests (ideally including both TSH and Free T4)
Calcium and phosphate
Creatine kinase, for evidence of muscle damage
Ferritin
IgA tissue transglutaminase antibodies (to exclude coeliac disease and assuming that the patient is not already on a gluten-free diet)
Urine dipstick (for blood protein and glucose)
The following tests are highly desirable, although not included in the NICE guidelines:
Vitamin D (especially in northern latitudes)
Iron, iron-binding capacity (transferrin saturation)
Vitamin B_{12}
Folate
Early morning cortisol (if there is a suspicion of Addison's disease)

Vitamin D deficiency increases muscular weakness if severe, and as many/most patients with ME/CFS and Long Covid tend to spend less time outside, vitamin D deficiency is increased in this group. However, studies of cohorts of ME/CFS patients have not shown overall that they have uniformly low levels compared to controls, although many patients had higher levels than controls because they were taking supplements. However, in unselected patients presenting with fatigue, vitamin D levels were reduced in 77% and the fatigue improved with supplemental vitamin D. Vitamin D deficiency is also commoner the further north one travels in the UK, so even if it is not the primary cause of fatigue, it may be a contributory cofactor that *is* amenable to treatment. Deficiencies of other vitamins and minerals may also be identified and may contribute to fatigue, even if they are not the primary cause.

In primary care, iron deficiency is usually detected by looking at a full blood count to assess haemoglobin and mean corpuscular volume (MCV). However, abnormalities in these are late changes. Ferritin is also used but the normal ranges usually quoted by laboratories are usually too low: above 15 is thought to indicate satisfactory iron levels, but studies have shown that a ferritin of at least 25 (and nearer 50) may be required to mitigate fatigue: this has been demonstrated in non-anaemic menstruating women. Measured ferritin may also be affected by any active inflammation; zinc protoporphyrin (ZPP) can be measured as an alternative that is not affected by inflammation. Raised ferritin, with fatigue, may be seen in the post-Covid syndrome, which may represent part of the initial hyper-inflammatory state. Sometimes very high ferritin levels are found which may indicate unsuspected haemochromatosis (especially in men and women post-menopause). If this is found further investigation and genetic testing may be appropriate. The highest levels of ferritin will be found in Still's disease (both childhood and adult-onset), where ferritin levels may be in the thousands.

The internet encourages people to believe that NHS thyroid function tests are inadequate. This is not true and NHS thyroid function tests are rigorously monitored by the laboratories and the laboratory performance is monitored UK-NEQAS and through inspections by UKAS. It has been reported that T3 levels are reduced and reverse T3 levels increased in some patients with ME/CFS. The significance of this is uncertain, but the finding was associated with other markers of low-grade inflammation, suggesting that the abnormalities may be part of a sick euthyroid syndrome, and not necessarily an indicator for thyroid replacement with either thyroxine or triiodothyronine.

There was a vogue for denying that tissue transglutaminase antibodies are better at diagnosing coeliac disease and associated neurological involvement (rare) than anti-gliadin antibodies. It is now accepted that this is incorrect and that anti-gliadin antibodies are less sensitive and less specific than tTG antibodies and there is no place for their measurement in routine clinical practice. tTG antibodies will disappear if the person is on a strict gluten-free diet, although this may take up to a year. tTG antibodies also provide a useful screen in known coeliacs for dietary compliance as the antibodies will either not disappear or will reappear if the diet contains gluten.

Abnormalities in the basic test results should always be further and appropriately investigated before confirming a diagnosis of ME/CFS.

The need for additional testing beyond those listed here should be identified from the history and examination. There is no value, with our current knowledge, in routine screening for infections, autoimmune disease, or endocrine disease without specific clinical indications. In primary care, this list comprises all that is necessary prior to referral to secondary care.

Common autoantibodies such as antinuclear antibodies have been reported in both ME/CFS and Long Covid, mainly in the early stages. These antibodies frequently occur in association with acute infections and will usually disappear fairly quickly. Adenovirus is particularly good at triggering antinuclear antibodies. Routine measurement, in the absence of features suggestive of a connective tissue disease such as Lupus, Sjogren's syndrome, or rheumatoid arthritis, is therefore unhelpful and may in fact be confusing if infection-triggered positives are identified.

Where Long Covid is suspected, it is crucial to verify evidence for infection with SARS-CoV2, rather than just assume that the chronic fatigue must be due to this. It may be appropriate to check basic clotting studies and look for anti-cardiolipin antibodies and lupus anti-coagulant (dRVVT), as abnormalities in clotting have been described in this condition, which may be linked to some of the early changes on MRI scans of the brains of patients with Long Covid. There has been very little research on clotting disorders in ME/CFS, but one recent study has identified similar abnormalities in ME/CFS to those found in Long Covid. If abnormalities are present, they may be present early in the course of the illness and have disappeared by the time the person eventually presents to a specialist, which may be months or even years down the line. Testing for anti-cardiolipin antibodies and lupus anti-coagulants in ME/CFS is only required if there is a history of a clotting disorder. Extensive livedo reticularis in the skin may be a visible marker of the anti-phospholipid syndrome.

There has been considerable research looking for a suitable diagnostic biomarker(s) for ME/CFS. This has not been terribly productive. There is still no single marker with a diagnostically useful sensitivity and specificity for ME/CFS. Panels of markers, mainly inflammatory cytokines, have been suggested as helpful, but these are not routinely available on the NHS and currently are more valuable in characterizing populations for research studies. It has been suggested that the combination of autoantibodies to β2-adrenoreceptors and M4 acetylcholine receptors, together with measurement of HHV6 levels, have diagnostic value, but the universal utility (and routine availability!) of these tests remains unproven at present.

Abnormalities on MRI, PET scanning, and electroencephalograph (EEG) have been reported in research trials and may be useful in phenotyping patients for research studies, but the changes are not sufficiently unique to allow the investigations to be used for diagnostic purposes. Routine use outside of trials is therefore not recommended unless there are findings on the history and examination which give rise to the suspicion of alternative diagnoses for which scanning is merited.

Postural orthostatic tachycardia syndrome (POTS) and vasovagal syncope are common in ME/CFS and a simple active stand test is helpful. Further investigations and advice on management if POTS is suspected should be obtained from an experienced physician. Phaeochromocytoma and cardiac rhythm abnormalities may present as POTS-like symptoms, so careful evaluation of the potential differential diagnosis is required.

FURTHER READING

Bansal, A.S. Investigating unexplained fatigue in general practice with a particular focus on CFS/ME. *BMC Fam Pract.* 2016;**17**:81. *https://doi.org/10.1186/s12875-016-0493-0.*

Roy S, Sherman A, Monari-Sparks MJ, Schweiker O, Hunter K. Correction of low vitamin D improves fatigue: effect of correction of low vitamin D in fatigue study (EViDiF Study). *N Am J Med Sci.* 2014;**6**(8):396–402. *https://doi.org/10.4103/1947-2714.139 291.*

Ruiz-Núñez B, Tarasse R, Vogelaar EF, Janneke Dijck-Brouwer DA, Muskiet FAJ. Higher prevalence of 'low T3 syndrome' in patients with chronic fatigue syndrome: a case-control study. *Front Endocrinol (Lausanne).* 2018;**9**:97. *https://doi.org/10.3389/fendo.2018.00097.*

Vaucher P, Druais PL, Waldvogel S, Favrat B. Effect of iron supplementation on fatigue in nonanemic menstruating women with low ferritin: a randomized controlled trial. *CMAJ.* 2012;**184**(11):1247–54. *https://doi.org/10.1503/cmaj.110950.*

CHAPTER 3

3.4 The dangers of diagnostic labels

Patients are very keen on diagnostic labels, but once applied, they become almost impossible to remove. Accordingly, it is crucial that a label of ME/CFS or Long Covid should not be applied unless there is clear evidence that the diagnostic criteria are met and that there is no possibility of a confounding illness. Patients may have increased anxiety when given a label of ME/CFS, fuelled by media misinformation: in these circumstances giving a diagnostic label early may increase symptoms. In the cases of uncertainty, a period of watchful waiting and regular re-evaluation is required. Patients do however have an expectation that the doctors in the medical assessment service will be able to give them a clear diagnosis and management plan, so managing this expectation is clearly an important part of a holistic approach to care. Patients need to have a clear understanding of the nature of their illness to be able to move on and adapt to living with it. Leaving the attribution of a diagnosis too long tends to lead to increased patient anxiety, often manifested by seeking further medical opinions, and delays the eventual acceptance of the diagnosis that is essential for moving forward.

In some cases, patients may have self-diagnosed as ME/CFS (via internet searches, books, alternative practitioners), and become frustrated with a process that challenges their assumptions. This must be handled with tact and empathy. Explaining that nearly half of patients presenting to a specialist clinic with 'chronic fatigue' turn out to have other medical problems is helpful. One of my early cases was convinced he had ME/CFS and was bullied into coming to the clinic by his wife, who was fed up with his longstanding ill-health. He turned out to have Addison's disease, with undetectable cortisol. Despite appropriate therapy, his fatigue improved only very slowly, presumably because of the very long duration of hypocortisolism.

Once a patient has acquired a label of chronic fatigue (or any other chronic diagnosis) there is a medical and patient tendency to subsequently attribute any new symptoms to the existing diagnosis. From the medical perspective this leads to a failure to apply proper diagnostic skills of taking new history and completing an appropriate physical examination and being prepared to investigate afresh. This is extremely dangerous and may lead to coincidental serious pathology being missed. All new symptoms in patients with ME/CFS and Long Covid should be investigated on their merits. Examples from personal experience of patients referred to a ME/CFS clinic include subsequent diagnoses of rheumatoid arthritis on more than one occasion, where there was no evidence of this at the original consultation and inflammatory markers were normal, and temporal arteritis in an older patient with very longstanding ME/CFS, where the increased headache was blamed on worsening of the ME/CFS: he had very elevated inflammatory markers. If symptoms change, the diagnosis should always be reviewed. Remember that a diagnosis of ME/CFS is based on a set of criteria and normal blood tests at one particular point in time. Having ME/CFS does not exclude the person getting other unrelated illnesses as time progresses. Particular red flags are: new swelling of joints; unilateral neurological symptoms; sudden change in bowel habit; new central chest pain related to exercise, among others.

Guidelines on the diagnosis of ME/CFS in children, adolescents, and adults are available in the UK through NICE and have been published in USA and Europe, as discussed. However, a structured approach, to history, examination, and investigation is crucial to ensuring that patients get the correct diagnosis and then the correct treatment.

CHAPTER 3

Primary ME/CFS or Long Covid versus secondary chronic fatigue

---

KEY POINTS

- Both ME/CFS and Long Covid may present as mild, moderate, or severe illnesses.
- There is a very long list of other medical and psychiatric conditions that may cause secondary chronic fatigue. Most of these will be identified by careful history, examination, and basic blood tests.
- Specific scoring tests may be helpful to identify some specific secondary causes such as sleep apnoea.

ME/CFS is strongly associated with related syndromes such as fibromyalgia, postural orthostatic tachycardia syndrome, and vasovagal syncope.

4.1 Spectrum of illness

Although diagnostic criteria have been laid down, every patient is different to a certain extent. Part of the skill of the experienced Fatigue Specialist is being able to identify deviations from the standard presentation that might give clues to other illnesses or conditions. This requires a broad knowledge and experience of general medicine. One of the issues with medicine now is that it is increasingly specialized and that specialization takes place much earlier in the doctor's career than it used to do. When I started training, most doctors, apart from a few specialists in teaching hospitals, would regard themselves as 'general physicians', doctors who could see any patient with a non-surgical condition make a reasonable attempt at a diagnosis, initiate treatment, and if concerned seek a second opinion from a specialist physician. As medicine has become increasingly complex, this type of doctor has gradually disappeared. 'General medicine' now simply refers to doctors who take part in acute unselected medical admissions, but even these have now evolved into 'acute physicians' who are specialists in the diagnosis and treatment of the acutely ill. While this is in itself a desirable change, the disappearance of general physicians in the routine outpatients is not. The Chief Medical Officer for England, Professor Sir Chris Whitty, has himself made a plea for the return of generalists, especially in care of older people. GPs now have nowhere to send patients where it is not immediately clear what organ specialty is most appropriate. Depending on the presenting symptoms, this can lead to a merry-go-round of referrals to different specialities, each of which undertakes a range of specialist tests before concluding that there is no evidence for a problem attributable to their '-ology' and referring the disillusioned patient back to the GP to refer on to a different specialty. This is a very expensive way of progressing a diagnosis as the patient has multiple clinic attendances and many investigations, some or all of which are unnecessary. Patients get understandably very frustrated by this, which encourages self-referral to individuals or services outside of the NHS, which may or may not be helpful, depending on the skills and experience of the practitioners concerned.

The wide variety of symptoms in patients with chronic fatigue creates a dilemma for even the best GP as to where the patient should be referred for appropriate investigation and management. This assumes of course that the GP and specialists do not simply take the negative investigations from the different '-ologies' as indicating that there is nothing wrong and inappropriately labelling the illness as purely psychological, or worse, factitious (not uncommon!).

Quite a number of the UK fatigue specialists have been immunologists. While there are increasing pointers that the cause of ME/CFS is immunological, in the past their involvement was more prosaically due to the fact that no one understood immunology, so if you had a patient with unexplained symptoms then you would refer to an immunologist because you had no idea what they did! Curiously, many recruits into immunology had unusual backgrounds in other medical specialities before switching to immunology. My training included spells in gastroenterology, chest medicine, and infectious diseases, as well as lots of acute emergency medicine! This was clearly helpful. Infectious disease specialists are also commonly involved in the assessment of patients with ME/CFS. Because of the predominance of lung problems in acute COVID-19 infection, respiratory physicians have frequently been involved in the management of Long Covid. Despite the existence of ME/CFS services in most areas of England, these were not used initially for Long Covid, although with time and the appreciation of the alignment of Long Covid with CFS/ME, the pathways are sensibly being merged.

The diagnostic criteria give a starting place for evaluating patients. (See previous chapter.) However, ME/CFS overlaps with a number of other related illness presentations, all of which include debilitating fatigue as a component, such fibromyalgia, irritable bowel syndrome, irritable bladder syndrome, POTS (postural orthostatic hypotension syndrome), and DEMS (dry eye and mouth syndrome), which are discussed next. See Figures 4.1 and 4.2.

ME/CFS, while consistent in the range of symptoms, may differ in its presentation in the early stages. Some patients have pure chronic fatigue, with little in the way of other symptoms, while at the other end of the spectrum, there are patients with fatigue and marked fibromyalgic pain symptoms (Figure 4.2). The majority of patients, however, fall somewhere in between the two extremes, with varying levels of fatigue and pain. Over the longer term, patients may move backwards and forwards between the two extremes. Patients' symptoms

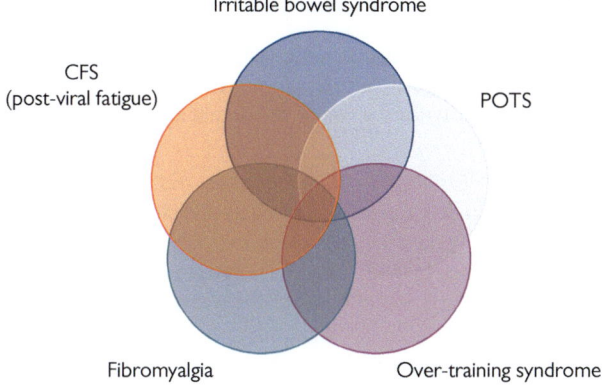

Figure 4.1 Overlap of fatigue syndromes.

may not be static either and typical ME/CFS symptoms which are not present at the outset may develop later and symptoms initially present may disappear and then reappear, especially if there are relapses. As noted in the previous chapter, this means that changes in patients' symptoms need to be carefully reviewed.

The NICE Guideline (ng206) provides advice on categorizing the severity of ME/CFS (see Box 4.1). This is useful for categorizing severity. There are also additional considerations in the section in Box 4.1 on care for people with severe or very severe ME/CFS. Definitions of severity are not clear-cut because individual symptoms vary widely in severity and people may have some symptoms more severely than others. The following definitions provide a guide to the level of

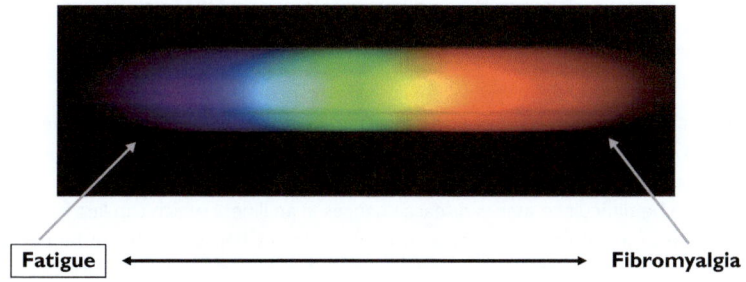

CFS/ME form a spectrum with varying degrees of pain and fatigue

Figure 4.2 Spectrum of fatigue and fibromylagic pain.

CHAPTER 4

Box 4.1 NICE Classification of severity of ME/CFS

NICE guidance is prepared for the National Health Service in England. All NICE guidance is subject to regular review and may be updated or withdrawn. NICE accepts no responsibility for the use of its content in this product/publication.

Mild ME/CFS

People with mild ME/CFS care for themselves and do some light domestic tasks (sometimes needing support) but may have difficulties with mobility. Most are still working or in education, but to do this they have probably stopped all leisure and social pursuits. They often have reduced hours, take days off, and use the weekend to cope with the rest of the week.

Moderate ME/CFS

People with moderate ME/CFS have reduced mobility and are restricted in all activities of daily living, although they may have peaks and troughs in their level of symptoms and ability to do activities. They have usually stopped work or education, and need rest periods, often resting in the afternoon for 1 or 2 hours. Their sleep at night is generally poor quality and disturbed.

Severe ME/CFS

People with severe ME/CFS are unable to do any activity for themselves or can carry out minimal daily tasks only (such as face washing or cleaning teeth). They have severe cognitive difficulties and may depend on a wheelchair for mobility. They are often unable to leave the house or have severe and prolonged after-effects if they do so. They may also spend most of their time in bed and are often extremely sensitive to light and sound.

Very severe ME/CFS

People with very severe ME/CFS are in bed all day and dependent on care. They need help with personal hygiene and eating, and are very sensitive to sensory stimuli. Some people may not be able to swallow and may need to be tube-fed.

impact of symptoms on everyday functioning. It is helpful to grade the severity of symptoms at the start of the illness: this can be repeated at intervals as required. The same structure can be used to look at the severity of Long Covid.

It can be difficult to assess disease changes in an illness which can last for years. The use of a simple functional questionnaire (see Chapter 14.2) can be helpful. There are many complex scoring systems for ME/CFS that are used primarily for research purposes, but these are often unwieldy for routine clinical use, e.g. De Paul Questionnaire (Bedree et al., 2019). In the UK, scoring systems were recommended by NICE in the original guidelines for assessment of ME/CFS (with appropriate permissions granted for copyright material). The purpose of these was to ensure that a standardized data set was collected. Centres have added other scoring systems as time has passed to address other issues. These originally included: HADS; Chalder Fatigue Score; Visual Analogue Pain Rating Scale; Self-Efficacy Scale; SF-36; EQ5D; and Epworth Sleep Score. Other scoring systems, for example, the Beighton score for hypermobility and scoring systems for autonomic dysfunction and autism (AQ-10), can also be used, as appropriate. These can also be applied to patients with Long Covid. Therapy services will often use a range of simple scores to assess patients before, during and at the end of therapeutic interventions and may repeat the main scoring systems to fully assess benefit (or lack of it). Often while the scores do not change much, the patient's perception of their illness can change dramatically as a result of interventions, which highlights the weakness of scoring systems compared against patients' own perceptions.

FURTHER READING

Bedree H, Sunnquist M, Jason LA. The DePaul symptom questionnaire-2: a validation study. *Fatigue*. 2019;7(3):166–79. *https://doi.org/10.1080/21641846.2019.1653471*.

Fisk JD, Ritvo PG, Ross L, Haase DA, Marrie TJ, Schlech WF. Measuring the functional impact of fatigue: initial validation of the fatigue impact scale. *Clin Infect Dis*. 1994;18 Suppl 1:S79–83. *https://doi.org/10.1093/clinids/18.supplement_1.s79*.

4.2 Secondary causes of fatigue

4.2.1 Introduction

Fatigue is not unique to ME/CFS and, in the grand scheme of things, other medical conditions must be considered and excluded before a diagnosis of ME/CFS is made. This chapter is therefore extremely important for the physician assessing any patient presenting with chronic fatigue. The differential diagnosis is extensive and requires familiarity with a wide range of conditions. The diagnostic tests described in the previous chapter will identify many (but not all!) of the other causes of fatigue. Fatigue is a common symptom in many if not all chronic illnesses. Patient self-diagnosis with ME/CFS without proper evaluation by a doctor is unwise if not dangerous. While at the moment there is no specific curative treatment for ME/CFS or Long Covid, many of the other conditions that may mimic ME/CFS and Long Covid ARE treatable.

4.2.2 Vitamin and mineral disorders

4.2.2.1 *Iron deficiency*

Deficiency of iron (ferritin <20 mcg/L) may cause fatigue even if the haemoglobin is not significantly reduced. A low MCV (mean corpuscular volume) may be an indicator on the screening full blood count and should be investigated with serum iron and ferritin (transferrin saturation and zinc protoporphyrin may also be used). Ferritin is an acute phase reactant (it goes up if there is inflammation) and will be elevated in line with C-reactive protein. Many laboratories report an inappropriate lower limit of normal for ferritin, which causes confusion. A diagnosis of ME/CFS should not be made until the patient is fully iron replete (with a ferritin above 25 mcg/L) and symptoms have been documented not to have improved. Low iron may also be a symptom of bowel disease and failure to absorb the mineral, for example coeliac disease (see next). It is important to identify why iron stores are low, for example inadequate intake, poor absorption (too much tea!), primary bowel disease, or excessive loss.

FURTHER READING

Vaucher P, Druais PL, Waldvogel S, Favrat B. Effect of iron supplementation on fatigue in nonanemic menstruating women with low ferritin: a randomized controlled trial. *CMAJ.* 2012;184(11):1247–54. *https://doi.org/10.1503/cmaj.110950.*

4.2.2.2 *Folate and B_{12} deficiency*

Severe deficiency of folic acid and vitamin B_{12} will cause anaemia: both cause a raised MCV. Both may be due to dietary deficiency. Vitamin B_{12} deficiency may also be caused by an autoimmune condition, pernicious anaemia, with antibodies against gastric parietal cells and intrinsic factor (a protein secreted by the stomach that is essential for binding vitamin B_{12} and transporting it to the terminal ileum at the end of the small intestine) where it is absorbed. Genetic deficiency of transcobalamin, required for blood transport of the vitamin, will also cause severe deficiency. The screening full blood count should identify these deficiencies as a potential cause of fatigue. There is a school of thought that vitamin B_{12} therapy, even if levels are normal, is advantageous in ME/CFS (see drug treatment Section 8.13).

4.2.2.3 *Vitamin D deficiency*

Vitamin D deficiency may cause fatigue, muscle weakness, and bone pain. Vitamin D is essential for calcium uptake from the bowel. Up to 30% of the population in the North of England may be vitamin D deficient due to lack of sun exposure during the summer. People who avoid the sun because of skin conditions or use high-factor sunblock creams are also at risk. As this is a treatable cause of fatigue, it is wise to check vitamin D levels and ensure replacement. Levels <25 ng/ml may be associated with symptoms.

Longstanding ME/CFS and Long Covid patients who are housebound are at risk of secondary vitamin D deficiency, which will worsen symptoms. Otherwise, unexplained deterioration of fatigue or new muscle weakness is an indication to recheck vitamin D levels.

4.2.3 Metabolic disorders

4.2.3.1 *Morbid obesity*

Under the Fukuda criteria, morbid obesity with a body mass index (BMI) >40 is an exclusion criterion for ME/CFS. Such patients will be fatigued and have significantly raised risk factors for other fatiguing comorbidities such as sleep apnoea, chronic cardiac disease, Type II diabetes, fatty liver, etc. Ideally, management should include weight loss via community-based management with an emphasis on dietetic input and assessment for drug therapy and gastric banding. Nonetheless, there may be some obese patients for whom a diagnosis of ME/CFS is appropriate, but the diagnosis is difficult.

4.2.3.2 *Diabetes mellitus*

Persistently raised blood sugar is associated with fatigue. This applies to undiagnosed diabetics and known diabetics with poor glucose control. It affects both Type I and Type II diabetics. In this context, it can be difficult to separate secondary and primary chronic fatigue until there is good diabetic control over a reasonable period. See section 4.2.5 on endocrine disorders.

4.2.3.3 *Calcium disorders*

Both hypocalaemia and hypercalcaemia are associated with fatigue. Hypocalaemia is associated with tetany and muscle weakness, while hypercalcaemia is associated with confusion and brain fog. Screening calcium levels in patients presenting with fatigue is therefore essential.

4.2.4 Gastrointestinal disorders

4.2.4.1 *Coeliac disease (unless there is evidence of good compliance with GFD, with negative tTG antibody)*

Untreated coeliac disease is a cause of chronic fatigue and this may be the only symptom. Coeliac disease is an immunological disorder where there is damage to the lining of the intestine which impairs the ability to digest food and absorb nutrients. The immunological reaction is triggered by the consumption of foods containing gluten, which is principally but not exclusively found in wheat. The screening of fatigued patients should always include a blood test for coeliac disease (antibodies to tissue transglutaminase (tTG)). If the test is positive, then further investigation by a gastroenterologist is necessary to confirm the diagnosis and to advise on treatment, in conjunction with a specialist dietician. A biopsy is no longer automatically required if the tTG antibodies are strongly positive, unless there is suspicion of complications. On a successful gluten-free diet symptoms will improve and the antibodies to tTG will gradually disappear. It may take 1–2 years for the fatigue to disappear completely, where the disease has been longstanding. It is essential that that the tTG (tissue transglutaminase) antibodies are monitored. These antibodies will disappear in GFD-compliant patients: if they are still present then there is gluten in the diet and the patient may still have active disease. Patients with known coeliac disease and good compliance should be assessed for ME/CFS on their individual merits, but with emphasis on a careful search for complications of coeliac disease (vitamin and mineral deficiencies, small bowel lymphoma). It is of course entirely possible to have both coeliac disease AND ME/CFS!

4.2.4.2 Inflammatory bowel diseases

Any form of occult inflammation is a risk factor for fatigue. The presence of gastrointestinal symptoms in conjunction with raised inflammatory markers (CRP and ESR) in a patient presenting with fatigue should raise the possibility that fatigue is secondary to inflammatory bowel disease.

4.2.4.3 Irritable bowel syndrome (IBS)

IBS symptoms are extremely common in primary chronic fatigue. Conversely, patients with a primary diagnosis of IBS are often fatigued. For patients presenting with prominent IBS symptoms, it is important to look for other key clinical features of chronic fatigue syndrome and not just focus on the management of the bowel disease. It is also important to ensure that other causes of bowel pathology have been excluded.

4.2.5 Liver disease

4.2.5.1 Haemochromatosis

Haemochromatosis, in which the body stores too much iron in the liver can present in the early stages with just fatigue. This is seen more often in men and postmenopausal women. Premenopausal women with regular periods lose enough iron each month to keep the symptoms at bay until menopause. As the disease progresses, diabetes develops, the skin develops a bronze discolouration due to the deposition of iron, and the liver is progressively damaged (cirrhosis). Arthritis occurs due to iron deposits in the joints. This is a genetic condition, so there may be a family history. In the beginning, the only blood abnormalities will be a very raised ferritin (in the absence of inflammation, as judged by CRP/ESR). As the disease progresses, the liver function tests (LFTs) become abnormal and the blood glucose rises. A genetic test is available. Treatment initially is by regular removal of blood, which mobilizes the iron from the liver. Other treatments are available from specialist centres.

4.2.5.2 Autoimmune liver disease

Primary biliary cirrhosis is an autoimmune liver disease, characterized by autoantibodies against mitochondrial antigens (anti-M2 antibodies). It is strongly associated even in the early stages with marked fatigue and autonomic symptoms. Chronic active (autoimmune) hepatitis, another autoimmune liver disease, with autoantibodies against smooth muscle (anti-actin autoantibodies), is not associated with fatigue, which is very curious and remains unexplained. Sclerosing cholangitis is another autoimmune disease, affecting the bile ducts, which is strongly associated with inflammatory bowel diseases, both ulcerative colitis and Crohn's disease. Significant fatigue, insomnia and sleep disturbances are frequently reported and may appear before other more obvious signs of bile duct damage are present.

Other forms of advanced chronic liver disease, such as alcoholic cirrhosis, will inevitably be accompanied by fatigue.

4.2.6 Endocrine disorders

4.2.6.1 New diagnosis or poorly controlled endocrine syndromes (diabetes, Addison's disease thyroid disease, PCOS)

Disturbance of the system of hormones in the body can cause significant fatigue. The basic blood screen recommended in the previous chapter will pick up the commonest hormonal problems such as diabetes and thyroid disease. Many of these conditions are immunologically linked, so for example patients with thyroid disease are more likely to get pernicious anaemia due to deficiency of vitamin B_{12}, caused by autoantibodies to gastric parietal cells and intrinsic factor. All may present with chronic fatigue.

Patients should not be diagnosed with ME/CFS if there is an untreated hormonal condition or until there is evidence of stable control of the metabolic/endocrine syndrome over a period of one year without resolution of fatigue. However, autoimmune endocrine disorders and ME/CFS are both relatively common and so can co-exist. If the fatigue persists, it is important to ensure that further investigation for associated illness is undertaken, for example coeliac disease in Type I diabetes, Addison's disease in patients with thyroid disease and pernicious anaemia with thyroid disease. For patients whose fatigue persists despite good control of the endocrine disorder, evaluation for ME/CFS should be undertaken in the normal way and referral to the therapy team considered if it is clear that there is no evidence for untreated medical disease. It is unhelpful to diagnose ME/CFS when underlying endocrine disorders are not stable on current management.

4.2.6.2 Thyroid disease

Because thyroid disease is common, the development of intercurrent thyroid disease in a patient with known chronic fatigue is not uncommon, but the diagnosis is often delayed because symptoms are attributed to a relapse of the CFS. Therapy with thyroxine (T4), or T3 or thyroid extracts in patients with normal thyroid function is suggested by some alternative practitioners as being valuable as treatment for ME/CFS. This is on the basis that NHS thyroid function tests do not reliably diagnose sub-clinical hypothyroidism and that thyroid extracts or triiodothyronine (T3) are better than standard thyroxine. There is however no scientific evidence to support the use of thyroid extracts, which are not standardized and do not give reliable control. Hypothyroidism due to pituitary failure will potentially be missed if thyroid-stimulating hormone (TSH) alone is used as a screening test. However, clinical history and examination should identify other features of pituitary insufficiency. Thyroid replacement is only indicated in patients with persistent biochemical evidence of hypothyroidism. Some patients do feel better with combined T4 and T3 replacement, even though the conventional advice is that T4 alone is satisfactory. Advice from a thyroid specialist should be sought if symptom control is poor with thyroxine alone or if dosing is difficult.

4.2.6.3 Addison's disease

Addison's disease, which is due either to immune destruction of the adrenal gland or to tuberculosis (the major cause worldwide), leads to a reduced production of the stress hormone cortisol and may present with fatigue to CFS/ME services. This may be difficult to diagnose clinically. Weight loss, nausea and non-specific malaise are additional features Pigmentation of non-sun-exposed areas (palmar creases, buccal mucosa) is highly suggestive. There may be postural hypotension. Electrolytes may show raised potassium and reduced sodium. Early morning cortisol will be low. A random cortisol >550 nmol/L excludes the diagnosis. There may be autoantibodies to adrenal antigens. If there is doubt, then a short synacthen test should confirm whether the adrenal gland is functioning normally. Adrenal failure may also arise as a consequence of tuberculosis, although this is rare in the UK, but should be considered in people from countries where TB is endemic.

4.2.6.4 Polycystic ovarian syndrome

Patients with polycystic ovarian syndrome (PCOS) may experience fatigue as part of the metabolic syndrome. This may be compounded by a raised BMI, which is a common feature. Some of the symptoms may be ameliorated by treatment, which should be initiated by a specialist. Chronic endometriosis is also associated with chronic fatigue.

4.2.6.5 Diabetes mellitus

Uncontrolled diabetes will cause fatigue. Type I, young onset, diabetes is immunologically based and is associated with other autoimmune conditions such as thyroid disease, Addison's disease, pernicious anaemia, and coeliac disease. If a Type I diabetic, who is well-controlled, develops persistent fatigue then it is important to check that there are no other linked autoimmune conditions present. Diabetics can still develop ME/CFS or Long Covid, so, provided that control is good, and there are no other associated conditions, it is entirely appropriate to consider these diagnoses.

Type II, late onset, diabetes is not an immunologically based condition but is linked more to diet and weight. If it is not well-controlled, then fatigue can be an issue.

4.2.7 Inflammatory arthritis (including early RA) and connective tissue diseases

In inflammatory arthritides and connective tissue diseases, the NICE recommended screening tests should identify evidence of raised inflammatory markers (C-reactive protein, CRP, and erythrocyte sedimentation rate, ESR). History and examination should identify specifically symptoms of morning stiffness and joint swelling. Anti-CCP antibodies are a more sensitive and specific test for early rheumatoid arthritis than rheumatoid factor, where there is a high pre-test probability. Fatigue may be the first presenting sign of rheumatoid arthritis, before there is very much in the way of joint pain or swelling. I have seen several cases over the years where patients that I thought had typical ME/CFS and who had normal inflammatory markers turned out months later to have typical features of rheumatoid arthritis, with positive blood markers and elevated inflammatory markers. This emphasizes the importance of re-evaluating people in whom a diagnosis of ME/CFS has been made but who develop new signs/symptoms. This includes repeating blood tests.

Fatigue is also a significant and often presenting feature in other connective tissue diseases such as systemic lupus erythematosus, Sjögren's syndrome, and seronegative arthritides (ankylosing spondylitis, psoriatic arthropathy, etc.). Sjögren's syndrome is very strongly associated with chronic fatigue. Dry eyes and mouth are typical and there are very specific autoantibodies present in the blood stream (anti-Ro and anti-La). DEMS mimics Sjögren's syndrome, but inflammatory markers are not elevated and the marker autoantibodies are absent. The fatigue will respond to the treatment of the underlying illness and the patient should be referred on to an appropriate specialist.

4.2.7.1 Vasculitis (inflammation in the blood vessels)

Vasculitis refers to inflammation in the blood vessels. There are a number of conditions, but the commonest and most likely to be confused with ME/CFS are giant cell arteritis (GCA, also known as temporal arteritis) and polymylagia rheumatic. In these conditions, the inflammatory markers in the blood (CRP and ESR) should be elevated. The platelet count is also usually increased. Careful consideration should be given to the possibility of polymyalgia rheumatica in the older population of patients presenting with 'fatigue', and of temporal arteritis in those presenting with fatigue and headache. Occasional patients with these conditions have normal inflammatory markers. While usually considered as disorders of older people (>60), both diseases may occur, albeit rarely, in patients in the age range 40–60, which can present diagnostic challenges. Diagnosis of GCA is assisted by temporal artery ultrasound and targeted biopsy. Vascular MRI and PET scanning may be valuable in defining more widespread vascular involvement and if there is suspicion of retinal involvement, then retinal angiography is essential. Both conditions respond well to treatment with corticosteroids with rapid resolution of symptoms. If the conditions are suspected but the inflammatory markers are normal, a trial of steroids is justified, but this may render biopsies and imaging inconclusive. If there is no response to steroids, then polymyalgia rheumatica or GCA are unlikely to be the cause of symptoms.

There are a range of other inflammatory conditions of the blood vessels but these are much rarer and have other very specific features.

4.2.8 Joint hypermobility (including Ehlers–Danlos syndrome)

Minor degrees of joint hypermobility are not uncommon. Many patients with confirmed ME/CFS have joint hypermobility. If the joint hypermobility is marked, particularly if there have been joint subluxations/dislocations, then it is worth considering a diagnosis of Ehlers–Danlos syndrome (EDS). This is a genetically based disorder, where there are defects in the genes for collagen and other closely related structural proteins in the musculoskeletal system. At least 19 different genetic variants are known and the disease can be both dominant or recessive. There are often complications affecting the skin, heart, eye, bowel, nervous system (due to joint problems at the base of the skull) and most other organ systems. Fatigue is a major feature and orthostatic intolerance is often present (POTS, vasovagal syncope, VVS). Management is complex, and patients with these disorders need multidisciplinary care, which is often lacking in the UK. Genetic testing will identify the majority of cases. However, some severe cases of hypermobile EDS have no currently identifiable genetic abnormality. There is no disease specific treatment at the present and management of the complications is all that can be offered. Because of the fatigue and the lack of alternative services, fatigued hypermobile EDS patients may be referred to ME/CFS services. Key management steps should include referral for genetic screening, screening for cardiac and valvular defects, and eye screening. Scanning of the neck may be necessary to identify subluxation of atlanto-occipital joint or the Arnold-Chiari malformation. Some patients have suggested that surgery to fix the Arnold-Chiari malformation has had a dramatic effect on their fatigue.

FURTHER READING

Hakim A, De Wandele I, O'Callaghan C, Pocinki A, Rowe P. Chronic fatigue in Ehlers–Danlos syndrome—hypermobile type. *Am J Med Genet C: Semin Med Genet.* 2017;175(1):175–80. *https://doi.org/10.1002/ajmg.c.31542.*

4.3 Allergy

Chronic allergic inflammation is usually accompanied by fatigue. Patients with perennial rhinosinusitis and/or conjunctivitis may present to chronic fatigue services. Headache, disturbed sleep, dizziness and fatigue are major features, in addition to localized nasal and eye symptoms. Fatigue may be exacerbated by daytime use of chlorphenamine (Piriton®), a sedating antihistamine. Some third-generation 'non-sedating' antihistamines may also cause sedation and dizziness in some patients.

Cognitive impairment may also be noted in patients on high-dose antihistamines. Chronic urticaria may also contribute to fatigue in its own right and be exacerbated by the need to use high-dose antihistamines to obtain control (often in doses 4x the normal recommended doses); therapy with anti-IgE monoclonal antibodies can provide significant benefit without the need for high doses of antihistamines, although the treatment is not curative and repeat courses may be required.

4.3.1 Mastocytosis

Mastocytosis, due to a clonal proliferation of mast cells, is associated with fatigue. Where the mast cells are present in the skin, they cause pigmented lesions (urticaria pigments), which urticate when scratched (Darier's sign). Systemic mastocytosis, where there is clonal proliferation of mast cells is in the bone marrow, can be harder to diagnose. Bone marrow involvement may be patchy and bone marrow biopsy may therefore miss the affected bone marrow. MRI of bones and bone marrow may identify affected areas and enable targeted biopsy. High-dose antihistamines used to control symptoms may increase fatigue. Biopsy of skin lesions and/or (targeted) bone marrow is usually diagnostic. Chemotherapy may be required.

4.3.2 Mast cell activation syndrome (MCAS)

There is a condition known as MCAS. The precise nature of this contain is uncertain but it is deemed to be distinct from mastocytosis, where clonal proliferation of mast cells can be identified. Typical features include marked fatigue, flushing, urticaria and angioedema, cognitive dysfunction, abdominal pain (often with diarrhoea), fibromyalgic pain, interstitial cystitis, joint hypermobility, headaches, autonomic dysfunction (POTS), and mood disorder. Clinical features, therefore, overlap with ME/CFS. It has been suggested that Long Covid may also be associated with features found in MCAS. There is no evidence of a clonal mast cell disorder (on bone marrow examination), and markers of mast cell activation (mast cell tryptase) may not be elevated, although there is debate as to whether this is the most appropriate test. It has been suggested that elevated plasma heparin may be more sensitive. Prostaglandins and leukotrienes, and chromogranin A have also been suggested as markers. Tests for specific allergies are usually negative. Management is often difficult.

FURTHER READING

Gülen T, Akin C, Bonadonna P, et al. Selecting the right criteria and proper classification to diagnose mast cell activation syndromes: a critical review. *J Allergy Clin Immunol Pract.* 2021;9(11):3918–28. *https://doi.org/10.1016/j.jaip.2021.06.011.*

Sumantri S, Rengganis I. Immunological dysfunction and mast cell activation syndrome in Long Covid. *Asia Pac Allergy.* 2023;13(1):50–3. *https://doi.org/10.5415/apallergy.00000 00000000022.*

4.4 Evidence of active chronic infection

Evidence of *active* chronic infection is an exclusion criterion for a diagnosis of chronic fatigue syndrome and patients should *not* be referred to therapy teams until it is clear that fatigue persists despite curative anti-infective therapy.

Fifty per cent of patients with ME/CFS have a sudden onset with an infective sounding illness. Unless patients are seen in the early phase (when it is not possible anyway to make a diagnosis of ME/CFS) aggressive investigation to identify the type of infection is not useful. Exceptions are those patients whose employment or social background puts them at risk of chronic infections (Lyme disease, Toxoplamosis, Brucellosis, TB), who should be investigated on merit. Fatigue is a common symptom of chronic hepatitis C (even in the absence of severe liver disease) and HIV infection. Patients with a history that could be consistent with possible contact with these viruses (intravenous drug use, use of anabolic steroid injections, sexual contacts with high-risk groups, multiple sexual partners) should be tested for these viruses and referred on to appropriate services if positive.

There is a perception in some groups of patients with ME/CFS that all CFS is due to a chronic variant of borreliosis (Lyme disease). Evidence to support this conclusion and the corollary that prolonged courses of antibiotics are helpful as a treatment for ME/CFS is lacking. This group of patients base their assumption on tests carried out outside the NHS, usually in the USA or Germany. It is important however to stress that Lyme disease, when properly diagnosed, is a potential cause of ME/CFS, but that this is a rare cause of ME/CFS in the UK. A persistent condition of post Lyme disease treatment syndrome (PLDT), with features similar to ME/CFS and Long Covid is seen in some patients after treatment for robustly confirmed acute Lyme disease.

As discussed in Chapter 1, there has historically been a lot of interest in enteroviruses as a potential cause of ME/CFS. The association of Long Covid with an acute viral infection has led to a resurgence of interest in enteroviruses as a potential trigger for ME/CFS, and newer diagnostic tests are now being applied to investigate this further (see Chapter 5.3).

Another popular view is that ME/CFS is due to chronic cytomegalovirus (CMV) infection, and that treatment with oral valganciclovir is appropriate. 40–60% of the population have evidence of CMV infection by the time they reach adulthood. Like other herpesviruses, once infected, CMV remains within the body and can be reactivated when the immune system is suppressed. The role of CMV in ME/CFS is not proven and valganciclovir, which is a toxic drug, is not justified without evidence of active current infection. If there is evidence of active CMV, as opposed to evidence of past infection, then referral to an infectious disease specialist is desirable.

Chronic Epstein–Barr virus infection (glandular fever) has also been suggested as a cause for ME/CFS and has a history in the USA (see Chapter 1). Most of the adult population have evidence of prior infection. It is therefore difficult to confirm that the virus is implicated, unless the person is investigated in the earliest stages of the illness, when IgM antibodies are detectable. CMV, EBV, HHV-6b, and HHV-7 and HSV (herpes simplex, cold sore virus) are all herpes viruses and once infected, the patient will continue to harbour the viruses in a latent form. The possible role of some of these viruses in the generation of ME/CFS is discussed in Chapter 5.3.

'Candida overgrowth' is a popular explanation advanced by patients for their fatigue, promoted by alternative practitioners. There is no convincing evidence for this, and the use of anti-fungals is not recommended in the absence of documented fungal infection. Anti-candida diets may improve irritable bowel-type symptoms in ME/CFS patients as they reduce the intake of resistant starches. Where there is severe and documented candida infection (positive cultures), chronic mucocutaneous candidiasis, which is an immune dysregulation syndrome, often with autoimmune endocrine features and having a genetic basis, should be considered. It is rare and typical features include oral and nail candidiasis: patients with these features should be referred to clinical immunology for formal evaluation.

FURTHER READING

Bai NA, Richardson CS. Posttreatment Lyme disease syndrome and myalgic encephalomyelitis/chronic fatigue syndrome: a systematic review and comparison of pathogenesis. *Chronic Dis Transl Med.* 2023;9(03):183–90. *https://doi.org/10.1002/cdt3.74.*

Brellier F, Pujades-Rodriguez M, Powell E, et al. (2022) Incidence of Lyme disease in the United Kingdom and association with fatigue: a population-based, historical cohort study. *PLoS ONE.* 17(3):e0265765. *https://doi.org/10.1371/journal.pone.0265765.*

4.5 Primary sleep disorders

Primary sleep disorders are usually distinguishable by virtue that the primary problem is not fatigue but inappropriate sleeping. Distinguishing between sleepiness and fatigue is therefore essential. All the primary sleep disorders have other specific features. Any such patients should be referred on to a specialist in sleep disorders (usually a neurologist) for further investigation and management. Referral to the ME/CFS Therapy teams is not appropriate.

4.5.1 Circadian rhythm disorder

This is a disorder usually seen in adolescents, where the body's natural clock becomes deranged, such that the person is awake all night and asleep all day (sleep reversal). It can be misdiagnosed as chronic fatigue, but the other associated features of ME/CFS are absent. It typically occurs in teenagers who spend a lot of time in the evening and at night on mobile phones and computers, as the blue light from these interferes with the normal stimuli to sleep; they often have limited exposure to natural daylight. Older people may also suffer from this, and triggers may be excessive coffee and/or alcohol consumption in the evening, drug abuse, and frequent air travel crossing multiple time zones. In adults, there are links to other neurological diseases, including Alzheimer's dementia, Huntington's disease, and Parkinson's disease, as well as strokes, conditions affecting vision (macula degeneration), and certain psychiatric conditions. It may also be seen in blind people. Management for young people is by avoiding triggers and a gradual reprogramming of bedtime and getting up times. Regular outdoor exercise is important, to ensure exposure to natural light. In older people, management is similar but there should be a search for underlying causes.

To complicate matters, circadian rhythm disorder may also occur as a *consequence* of ME/CFS and Long Covid.

FURTHER READING

Goldstein CA, Kagan D, Rizvydeen M, Warshaw S, Troost JP, Burgess HJ. The possibility of circadian rhythm disruption in Long Covid. *Brain Behav Immun Health*. 2022;**23**:100476. *https://doi.org/10.1016/j.bbih.2022.100476.*

4.5.2 Shift-worker's syndrome

This is a very particular form of a circadian rhythm disorder which occurs in people who work regular nightshifts over a long period of time. Young people can adapt reasonably to working nightshifts for a period, but in older people the adjustment to the body's natural clock (circadian rhythm) is not so well tolerated. Continuous nightshift working is actually easier to cope with than alternating day/evening/night shifts. Over time the compensatory mechanisms fail and sleep becomes very disordered, leading to a secondary and severe chronic fatigue. Obviously, management involves switching to a fixed shift pattern, or preferably doing day-only shifts. The resolution of the fatigue can be a very slow process. Melatonin may be helpful in the short term to re-establish a more normal sleep pattern.

FURTHER READING

Richter K, Acker J, Adam S, Niklewski G. Prevention of fatigue and insomnia in shift workers—a review of non-pharmacological measures. *EPMA J*. 2016;**7**(1):16. *https://doi.org/10.1186/s13167-016-0064-4.*

4.5.3 Narcolepsy

Narcolepsy may occasionally be mistaken for ME/CFS. The key clinical features are: excessive daytime sleepiness; sleep attacks (suddenly and inappropriately dropping off to sleep); cataplexy (sudden weakness often triggered by strong emotions); sleep paralysis on falling asleep or waking. Other features include hallucinations, headaches, and depression. Secondary narcolepsy may occur with MS, encephalitis, and head injury. In most cases, the cause appears to be due to interference with the hypocretin (orexin) pathway (not in all cases) and involves an autoimmune process against trib2 which impairs hypocretin production.

The major problem here is sleepiness not fatigue, which emphasizes the importance of distinguishing between the two (see 'What is fatigue', Chapter 2.1).

4.5.4 Restless legs (periodic limb movement disorder)

This condition is characterized by unpleasant sensations in the limbs accompanied by uncontrollable movements of the limbs, including in sleep. While it can occur by itself, it can be secondary to iron deficiency, chronic kidney disease, diabetes, Parkinson's disease, rheumatoid arthritis, and hypothyroidism, so it may also be linked to chronic fatigue.

4.5.5 REM Sleep behaviour disorder (RBD)

This is characterized by violent nightmares, often with dream enactment, which can lead to physical injury to the patient and partner. It is due to a failure of the normal voluntary muscular paralysis that occurs during rapid eye movement (REM) sleep. The dream enactment can be extremely frightening. Daytime fatigue and sleepiness results from the disturbed night-time sleep. It can be associated with Lewy body dementia, Parkinson's disease, and multiple system atrophy (MSA).

4.5.6 Idiopathic hypersomnia

This disorder is characterized by an excessive need for sleep, usually greater than 11 hours a day. The cause is unknown. Daytime grogginess and difficulty in waking are common. Difficulties are experienced in performing tasks and there is 'brain fog'. This condition can therefore cause confusion with ME/CFS. The use of sleep diaries can help.

4.5.7 Secondary sleep disorders (sleep deprivation)

Sleep deprivation with consequent daytime somnolence and fatigue may occur for example in mothers with children with sleep disturbance (night terrors, nocturnal head banging, etc.). Management of the underlying problem or the secondary cause may be required to solve the problem. This is not ME/CFS and management of the underlying cause of the sleep deprivation will, given time, resolve the daytime somnolence and fatigue. Sleep diaries may help to pinpoint the cause.

4.5.8 Obstructive sleep apnoea (OSA)

Sleep apnoea is commonly confused with ME/CFS, as the daytime symptoms are similar, with headache, sore throats, fatigue, and malaise. Pointers tend to be increased BMI, short neck, increasing collar size, or absolute collar size (17 or above), and evidence of a narrow pharynx with bulging side walls on inspection (this is scored using the Mallampati system: Grade III or IV is highly significant). The Epworth Sleep Score should be used and any patient with a score of 12 or above should be referred for sleep studies. The Epworth Sleep score is not infallible, and patients with symptoms but low scores may still have OSA, and conversely, those with raised scores may not be shown to have OSA on formal testing. Sleep apnoea is a risk factor for stroke and myocardial infarction. Patients with sleep apnoea who do not respond well to optimized CPAP (continuous positive airway pressure) should be evaluated for ME/CFS (they can co-exist!). Referral to a therapy team should not take place until there has been an effective trial of CPAP. Surgery is occasionally required to refashion the pharynx. Early phase trials are underway in the USA of a combination of the drugs aroxybutinin (used to treat overactive bladder symptoms) and atomoxetine (used to treat ADHD), which show apparent benefit. This will help those who are unable to tolerate CPAP.

For the sleep disorders mentioned, it may be appropriate to get patients to complete a sleep diary.[1]

4.5.8.1 *Neurological disease*

If there is any suspicion of neurological disease in a patient presenting with chronic fatigue, assessment by a neurologist is advisable.

4.5.9 Multiple sclerosis

The most important neurological disorder to consider is multiple sclerosis. This is an immune-mediated brain disease. Fatigue can be a prominent feature of chronic MS and may be an early feature. It is often accompanied by excessive daytime sleepiness and may be improved by activity, in contrast to ME/CFS. Usually, the history includes neurological symptoms occurring in different anatomical locations at different times. Where there is doubt, review by a neurologist should be obtained.

FURTHER READING

Broch L, Simonsen CS, Flemmen HØ, Berg-Hansen P, Skardhamar Å, Ormstad H, Celius EG. High prevalence of fatigue in contemporary patients with multiple sclerosis. *Mult Scler J Exp Transl Clin.* 2021;7(1):2055217321999826. *https://doi.org/10.1177/20552 17321999826.*

Torres-Costoso A, Martínez-Vizcaíno V, Reina-Gutiérrez S, et al. Effect of exercise on fatigue in multiple sclerosis: a network meta-analysis comparing different types of exercise. *Arch Phys Med Rehabil.* 2022;103(5):970–87. *https://doi.org/10.1016/ j.apmr.2021.08.008.*

4.5.10 Parkinson's disease and Parkinsonian syndromes

In older patients, Parkinson's disease (a neurological disorder due to dopamine depletion) may present primarily with fatigue, before the other more typical signs of gait abnormalities and tremor (typically described as 'pill-rolling'). Watching a patient get out of a chair and walk is key part of the examination: there may be a

---

[1] An example can be found at: *https://thesleepcharity.org.uk/wp-content/uploads/The-Sleep-Charity-Sleep-Diary.pdf*

delay in initiating walking, the gait may appear stiff and arm swing may be reduced. The face may be expressionless. Tremor may be present in ME/CFS but is usually sporadic, coarse, and easily stopped by distraction.

FURTHER READING

Lin I, Edison B, Mantri S, et al. Triggers and alleviating factors for fatigue in Parkinson's disease. *PLoS One*. 2021;16(2):e0245285. *https://doi.org/10.1371/journal.pone.0245285*.

4.5.11 Dementia

Patients with early Alzheimer's disease may also present to chronic fatigue clinics with marked fatigue. Features of concern would include predominance of memory problems (particularly short term, with preservation of long-term memory), loss of navigational skills (getting lost going to shops), and unexplained deterioration in work performance. However, most of these symptoms may also be seen in patients with ME/CFS and Long Covid, especially in the more severe forms. If there is doubt, then formal assessment in a dementia clinic is advised, as there are now treatments that may benefit some types of dementia in the early stages. Dementia with Parkinsonian features of tremor may suggest more severe diseases such as MSA or dementia with Lewy bodies. Both of these conditions may be accompanied by REM sleep disorder, where violent and vivid dreams are acted out by the patient while asleep (see earlier).

Studies on patients with Alzheimer's dementia who were infected with COVID-19 have shown a rapid acceleration of the disease. Although not proven it is feared that the neuroinflammatory aspects of ME/CFS and Long Covid may accelerate the development of Alzheimer's in those who have a predisposition to develop the illness.

Problems of memory in patients with ME/CFS and Long Covid can sometimes lead to unjustified fear of a diagnosis of dementia.

4.5.12 Chronic traumatic encephalopathy

There is increasing recognition of chronic traumatic encephalopathy (CTE) following head injury. Contact sports of direct blows to the head are the most common causes, but it can also be seen after rapid acceleration/deceleration or rotation of the head. While in most cases symptoms are transient after injury, they may become persistent, particularly in individuals with repeated injury (sports people). Typical symptoms include headaches, dizziness, fatigue, aversion to noise and light, blurred vision, neck pains, depression and anxiety, memory problems, brain fog, insomnia, and alcohol intolerance. All of these symptoms of course may be seen in ME/CFS and Long Covid. CTE may progress to a dementia-like illness. Checking patients presenting for the first time with chronic fatigue for a history of contact sports or head injuries is therefore important, before labelling them as ME/CFS. If CTE is suspected, a referral to a neurologist is advised.

FURTHER READING

Pierre K, Dyson K, Dagra A, Williams E, Porche K, Lucke-Wold B. Chronic traumatic encephalopathy: update on current clinical diagnosis and management. *Biomedicines.* 2021;9(4):415. *https://doi.org/10.3390/biomedicines9040415.*

4.5.13 Post Guillain–Barré syndrome

Chronic fatigue has also been noted in patients who have recovered from Guillain–Barré syndrome (GBS). As GBS is usually infection-driven and autonomic dysfunction is a well-recognized feature in the acute phase, it is not unreasonable to consider fatigue in this context as being identical to ME/CFS and appropriate to refer for therapy. Fatigue is also seen in chronic demyelinating neuropathies, but here there is an active inflammatory process that is usually undergoing active management.

FURTHER READING

de Vries JM, Hagemans ML, Bussmann JB, van der Ploeg AT, van Doorn PA. Fatigue in neuromuscular disorders: focus on Guillain–Barré syndrome and Pompe disease. *Cell Mol Life Sci.* 2010;67(5):701–13. *https://doi.org/10.1007/s00018-009-0184-2.*

4.5.14 Post-MI/stroke syndromes

Patients who have had major coronary events with arrest or peri-arrest situations often have suffered a degree of cerebral hypoxia, which causes fatigue, poor memory, and concentration and this is often accompanied by severe depressive illness, especially in younger males who lose their jobs as a result, or where the illness came out of the blue. Good cardiac rehabilitation may help. Symptoms typical of PTSD may also occur. ME/CFS therapy is unlikely to help as this is a neurological insult which will recover only slowly. Psychological input through community psychology services or through cardiac rehabilitation services is most appropriate. Similar problems are seen in patients post-stroke and are likely to increase as more patients undergo thrombolysis and have less residual motor deficit.

4.5.15 Chronic migraine

Chronic migraine is usually defined as migraine episodes on more than 15 days in each month. This can be extremely debilitating and also extremely fatiguing. Indeed, it is ranked in the top 40 of most debilitating chronic conditions world-wide. Needless to say, fatigue can be a serious component of the illness The diagnosis can be difficult and exclusion of other causes of chronic headache need to be excluded, especially if there has been a recent change in headache pattern. Referral to a headache or migraine clinic is advisable if this diagnosis is suspected, as there are a range of new hospital-only treatments available which can be very successful. Control of the migraine will usually improve the fatigue.

FURTHER READING

Karsan N, Goadsby PJ. Migraine is more than just headache: is the link to chronic fatigue and mood disorders simply due to shared biological systems? *Front Hum Neurosci.* 2021;15:646692. *https://doi.org/10.3389/fnhum.2021.646692.*

4.5.16 Epilepsy

Epilepsy is associated with fatigue. The more severe the epilepsy, the greater the risks of chronic fatigue. This may be most marked after fits but may also persist between fits. Medication used to treat epilepsy may also be contributory. It is of course possible to have both ME/CFS and epilepsy, and it can be hard to determine whether the CFS is primary or secondary to the epilepsy. A review of fit control and medication is appropriate before labelling the fatigue as primary ME/CFS.

FURTHER READING

Hamelin S, Kahane P, Vercueil L. Fatigue in epilepsy: a prospective inter-ictal and post-ictal survey. *Epilepsy Res.* 2010;91(2–3):153–60. *https://doi.org/10.1016/j.eplepsy res.2010.07.006.*

4.5.17 Pesticide poisoning

There are case reports of organophosphate and organochlorine pesticides causing a syndrome very similar to ME/CFS, with prolonged debilitating cognitive impairment. Mostly, exposure causes a severe acute syndrome, but for those that survive there may be a chronic debilitating illness. Chronic neuroinflammation is postulated to occur, which is a similar hypothesis to that currently being proposed in ME/CFS and Long Covid (see Chapter 5.4). Epilepsy may also occur. A good history should identify those at risk of this syndrome, mainly those working in the agricultural setting. Improvements in health and safety, together with a trend to reduce the use of such compounds, means that this is now rare in the UK.

FURTHER READING

Andrew PM, Lein PJ. Neuroinflammation as a therapeutic target for mitigating the long-term consequences of acute organophosphate intoxication. *Front Pharmacol.* 2021;12:674325. *https://doi.org/10.3389/fphar.2021.674325*

Richardson J. Four cases of pesticide poisoning, presenting as ME, treated with a choline and ascorbic acid mixture. *J Chronic Fatigue Synd.* 2000;6(2):11–21. *https://doi.org/ 10.1300/J092v06n02_03*

4.5.17.1 *Psychiatric disorders, including factitious illness*

It is important to consider psychiatric illness in all patients presenting with fatigue. Sometimes it is difficult to work out whether the problem is a primary depressive illness complicated by secondary fatigue or a primary fatigue complicated by secondary depression. There may be an overlap between depression, anxiety and ME/CFS which can make diagnosis difficult. One-third of patients with ME/CFS have comorbid depression. There are scoring systems such as the HADS for checking for depression, but none of them specifically identify whether the depression caused the fatigue or vice versa! If there is doubt, formal evaluation by an experienced psychologist or liaison psychiatrist should be sought prior to making a diagnosis of ME/CFS.

Either way if there is significant depression then treatment may be appropriate. If the depression is the cause of the fatigue then there may be some improvement in the fatigue with treatment. If the depression is secondary to ME/CFS, then treatment of the fatigue with appropriate supportive therapies may reduce the depression and parallel treatment of the depression may also help improve (but not cure the fatigue). A trial of anti-depressants for 4–6 months may be appropriate, but treatment may need to be extended. SSRIs (selective serotonin reuptake inhibitors) are the preferred drugs, although fluoxetine and paroxetine may be poorly tolerated in patients with ME/CFS; citalopram and venlafaxine seem to be better tolerated, although the latter should only be used with specialist advice.

It is important to identify patients whose fatigue is secondary to a primary psychiatric disorder, usually depression. Such patients will have the cardinal feature of low mood, with other symptoms such as loss of interest, loss of pleasure, loss of confidence, self-reproach or guilt, agitation, or retardation, as well as reduced concentration, change in appetite and sleep. There may be a diurnal variation of symptoms, including fatigue. Suicide risk needs to be explored. Where this is identified, patients should be referred to appropriate services for further management, unless there is immediate concern about suicide risk, in which case referral to the crisis team should be initiated.

4.5.18 Autistic spectrum disorders

Over the years, I have seen a number of patients presenting to the fatigue clinic where the diagnosis has turned out to be an autistic spectrum disorder. While most were teenagers, there were also adults whose condition was not diagnosed earlier in life. There is a recognized condition of autistic fatigue, where the stress of coping with sensory overload and social situations becomes too much. This can become severe: autistic burnout, with symptoms remarkably similar to ME/CFS. In general, patients with clearly diagnosed ME/CFS do not score more highly in tests for autistic spectrum disorders. It is important to recognize the possibility of an underlying autistic spectrum disorder in patients of any age presenting with fatigue. The AQ-10 score is a useful screen, but any suspected cases should be referred for formal and detailed evaluation, which may be difficult for adults as services are scarce/non-existent. NICE Guideline CG142 covers the diagnosis and management of autism in adults and children.

4.5.19 Factitious illness

Factitious or exaggerated illness, including Münchausen syndrome, is more difficult to identify without corroborative evidence from other sources. In children, the possibility of Münchausen by proxy may be considered. It is rare. If in doubt, seek advice from liaison psychiatry before diagnosing ME/CFS and initiating referral to therapy teams. Psychosomatic illness should also be considered. Symptom descriptions often include unusual symptoms, which may be lateralized, or which may be inconsistent with organic disease.

4.5.20 Eating disorders

Fatigue may be a presenting complaint of eating disorders, including anorexia, binge-eating disorder, bulimia, and orthorexia (eating a restricted diet to avoid eating 'unhealthy' foods). Very low body weight may give a pointer to anorexia, but the other conditions may be more difficult to detect without further direct questioning. Eating disorders are rarely admitted, especially anorexia. Confirmation from family and friends may be required. These conditions can lead to vitamin and mineral deficiencies, which contribute to fatigue, as well as other problems such as osteoporosis, and alkalosis due to repeated vomiting of acid stomach contents. Eating disorders are also associated with symptoms of POTS. The stress of ME/CFS and Long Covid may also lead to secondary eating disorders, as a way for the patient to achieve 'control' over their dysfunctional body. The relationship between eating disorders and fatigue is therefore complex. Managing one without the other is doomed to failure.

4.5.21 Post-traumatic stress disorder

A number of patients have been referred for medical assessment of fatigue where it is clear that the fatigue is part of a post-traumatic stress disorder. It is important in taking the history from a patient with suspected fatigue that major stressful events in the past are identified, especially in ex-military personnel. This must be done with sensitivity and often people may be reluctant to divulge highly personal events at the first consultation with a stranger. It is important to focus during history taking as the person may offer pointers that they want the doctor to ask further questions but do not want to spontaneously volunteer information. 'Is there anything else you want to tell me?' is an important question. Studies on ME/CFS patients show that they are more likely to report abuse in the past. Where this is identified, patients should be referred through their GP for appropriate counselling or primary care psychology and not to the chronic fatigue therapy teams. There are specific scoring systems for PSTD.[2]

4.5.22 School refusal

In teenagers, fatigue may form part of the spectrum of school refusal. It is important to investigate the educational background and social setting. School refusal may be linked to bullying at school or abuse.

---

[2] For more information, see: *https://www.ptsd.va.gov/professional/assessment/adult-sr/ptsd-checklist.asp*

FURTHER READING

Havik T, Ingul JM. How to understand school refusal. *Front Media SA*. 2021;6:715177. *https://doi.org/10.3389/feduc.2021.715177*.

4.5.23 Unexplained medical (neurological symptoms)

Fatigue may be a significant element in patients presenting with symptoms complexes which physicians are unable to match with known medical diseases. This is a particular problem in neurological disease. Some of these patients have unusual presentations of common or rare diseases or even new diseases but some clearly have psychosomatic or factitious illness. It is noteworthy that there appears to be a high incidence of unexplained neurological symptoms post-COVID-19 infection, although 90% of patients actually met the criteria for ME/CFS. Some of these will have a diagnosis of Long Covid. It is not however appropriate to put all patients with chronic fatigue or chronic pain into this category. Whatever the nature of the problem, these patients still require therapeutic input.

FURTHER READING

Husain M, Chalder T. Medically unexplained symptoms: assessment and management. *Clin Med (Lond)*. 2021;21(1):13–18. *https://doi.org/10.7861/clinmed.2020-0947*.

Kachaner A, Lemogne C, Dave J, Ranque B, de Broucker T, Meppiel E. Somatic symptom disorder in patients with post-COVID-19 neurological symptoms: a preliminary report from the somatic study (somatic symptom disorder triggered by COVID-19). *J Neurol Neurosurg Psychiatry*. 2022;93(11):1174–80. *http://dx.doi.org/10.1136/jnnp-2021-327 899*.

4.5.24 Fatigue related to other organ-specific disease (lung, heart, kidney) or its treatment

Fatigue as a consequence of chronic or sub-acute organ-based illness is common and its severity usually mirrors that of the primary disorder. Even moderate COPD (chronic obstructive pulmonary disease) is associated with significant fatigue and fatigue is actually the second most common symptom in COPD. Renal impairment is associated with fatigue at quite modest elevations of serum creatinine, well below those that would require renal treatment such as dialysis or transplantation. The fatigue in this setting is not ME/CFS. Where there is evidence for underlying chronic organ-based disease, the fatigue should be managed as part of the ongoing illness by the organ-based specialist.

FURTHER READING

Casillas JM, Damak S, Chauvet-Gelinier JC, Deley G, Ornetti P. Fatigue in patients with cardiovascular disease. *Ann Readapt Med Phys*. 2006;49(6):309–19, 392–402. *https://doi.org/10.1016/j.annrmp.2006.04.002*.

Ebadi Z, Goërtz YMJ, Van Herck M, et al. The prevalence and related factors of fatigue in patients with COPD: a systematic review. *Eur Respir Rev.* 2021;30(160):200298. *https://doi.org/10.1183/16000617.0298-2020.*

Gregg LP, Bossola M, Ostrosky-Frid M, Hedayati SS. Fatigue in CKD: epidemiology, pathophysiology, and treatment. *Clin J Am Soc Nephrol.* 2021;16(9):1445–55. *https://doi.org/10.2215/CJN.19891220.*

4.5.25 Fatigue secondary to malignancy and/or chemo/radiotherapy

Malignancy and chemo/radiotherapy for its treatment are all strongly associated with chronic fatigue, which may persist long term (5–30 years) even when the primary tumour has been fully treated. Breast and prostate cancer seem to be particularly associated with fatigue, but all malignancies can cause fatigue. Ninety per cent of patients with cancer report fatigue at some stage. It is important in medical screening of patients complaining of fatigue to be alert to the possibility of occult malignancy, seeking specifically evidence for unexplained localized symptoms/signs such as bone pain, new skin rashes, unexplained recurrent venous thrombosis, and other paraneoplastic phenomena. Depressive illness following a diagnosis of cancer is very common and will complicate matters. This is most appropriately dealt with through community psychology services. Palliative care services may also be able to advise on other avenues of support, as may cancer-specific patient support groups. Referral to ME/CFS therapy teams is unhelpful.

FURTHER READING

Thong MSY, van Noorden CJF, Steindorf K, Arndt V. Cancer-related fatigue: causes and current treatment options. *Curr Treat Options Oncol.* 2020;21(2):17. *https://doi.org/10.1007/s11864-020-0707-5.*

4.5.26 Gulf War syndrome

Gulf War syndrome was recognized after the conflict in the Middle East. Symptoms were very similar to ME/CFS, although significant organ damage seems to have been much more common. The precise cause has never been identified, despite various enquiries. It appeared to affect US and UK troops more than French troops. Suggested causes include side effects of the nerve gas prophylaxis (the French troops did not use this), low-grade exposure to nerve gases or depleted uranium (in artillery shells), and experimental vaccines or their adjuvants. Undoubtedly post-traumatic stress played a part in some cases, but not all.

FURTHER READING

James LM, Georgopoulos AP. At the root of 3 'long' diseases: persistent antigens inflicting chronic damage on the brain and other organs in Gulf War illness, Long Covid-19, and chronic fatigue syndrome. *Neurosci Insights.* 2022;17:26331055221114817. *https://doi.org/10.1177/26331055221114817.*

4.5.27 Burnout syndrome

The symptoms of burnout syndrome overlap with chronic fatigue. It is caused by chronic stress in the workplace and is characterized by exhaustion and deper- sonalization. It is most commonly seen in caring and social professions such as doctors, nurses, dentists, teachers, social workers and others working in public services (civil service). There has been a huge surge in this condition as a result of the extreme stress caused by the COVID-19 pandemic and the after-effect on waiting lists. Symptoms typically include chronic fatigue, chronic exhaustion, poor concentration and memory, loss of drive, personality changes, severe anx- iety and depression, and development of addictions. Physical symptoms can in- clude headaches, IBS, tachycardia, and arrythmia. Withdrawal in the workplace occurs and personal relationships at home are negatively affected. Long periods off work usually occur and premature attempts to return to work may lead to severe relapse. Identification of burnout is key as treatment requires focus on the working environment and working to improve stress management, relaxation, learning how to say 'No' and to delegate, and protecting 'me' time for hobbies and relaxation. The condition may be so severe that the affected person is unable to return to their employment.

FURTHER READING

Weber A, Jaekel-Reinhard A. Burnout syndrome: a disease of modern societies?. *Occup Med (Lond)*. 2000;**50**(7):512–17. *https://doi.org10.1093/occmed/50.7.512.*

4.5.28 Overtraining syndrome

The overtraining syndrome is recognized in sports medicine. The symptoms can mimic ME/CFS. It is usually seen in high-performance athletes but can be seen in recreational athletes who are training/racing too hard. As well as fatigue, there is usually marked sleep disturbance, increased resting heart rate, and deterior- ation of athletic performance. In patients presenting with fatigue it is therefore important to include inquiry about sports activity. Management should be centred on reducing training, increasing recovery time, and encouraging patience.

FURTHER READING

Armstrong LE, Bergeron MF, Lee EC, Mershon JE, Armstrong EM. Overtraining syndrome as a complex systems phenomenon. *Front Network Physiol*. 2022;1:20. *https://doi.org/ 10.3389/fnetp.2021.794392.*

4.6 Primary ME/CFS

Provided that the history is suggestive, blood tests have been unremarkable and there are no pointers to any other of the medical conditions discussed earlier that can also be associated with fatigue, it will be reasonable to make a diagnosis of chronic fatigue syndrome, ME/CFS. The criteria require the illness to have been present for months (at least four) before the diagnosis can be considered. This is unfortunate, although understandable. Experience suggests that the earlier the diagnosis is made and treatment instituted, the better the outcome. Delaying diagnosis for an arbitrary period of time also means that research into causation is prevented, as early abnormalities in blood tests or signs of acute infection will be missed.

Long Covid has been rather useful in this setting as patients have presented far earlier, and this has allowed acute investigation and then follow-up, giving a much better picture of the early stages of the development of chronic fatigue symptoms.

However, despite these advances, the diagnosis of ME/CFS remains one of exclusion. The more experienced the practitioner, the more likely it is that other potential causes of chronic fatigue will be identified. In my own clinic, the pick-up rate of alternative diagnosis was around 19% when I first started, but by the time I retired, the figure had risen to 47%. This of course was attributable to increasing awareness of fatigue in association with other conditions and liaising with colleagues in other disciplines. Equally, specialists in organ-based disciplines have become more aware of fatigue as a complication of organ-based illness and are more ready to seek second opinions.

History-taking from ME/CFS sufferers identifies two clear patterns of illness. One is a gradual onset, where there is no clear precipitating event, and the other is a very acute onset, with typical acute infectious symptoms that then do not resolve. Patients appear to divide with about a 50:50 split. In practice, it seems to make no difference to the long-term outcome and investigations when the patients reach a specialist clinic usually shows no material difference, but of course by the time the clinic is reached months have passed and any acute changes will have resolved and trying to identify a triggering infection in the acute onset group is impossible as too much time has passed. Very occasionally, there is evidence for infection, and this is not restricted to just viral infections: any type of acute infection can be a trigger, including bacteria. See section 4.1 and Chapter 5.3. Careful analysis of cohorts of ME/CFS patients can identify subgroups, based on clinical symptom clusters.

There has been a tendency in the past to try and label CFS and ME as different illnesses. This has largely been driven by the need for patients to have a clear diagnostic label, at a time when the medical profession was largely disbelieving. Most organizations now accept the term ME/CFS. Distinguishing ME/CFS from chronic fatigue as a secondary component of other illnesses remains important. Many doctors dislike the term myalgic encephalomyelitis, despite the fact that it originated from the medical profession after the Royal Free outbreak, but the fact that current research is pointing very directly to a neuroinflammatory brain disease suggests that the name may actually be very appropriate (see Chapter 5.4).

CHAPTER 4

The fact that there is a group with a very sudden infection-like onset is highly relevant when considering the impact that COVID-19 has had. In the past there has been a tendency to label the acute onset ME/CFS patients with a clear history of acute onset following infection, even if not confirmed by tests, as post-infectious chronic fatigue or post-viral chronic fatigue. This term is best reserved for cases where there has been an identifiable acute infection (Long Covid is a prime example). The fact that there is an identifiable acute infection seems to make little difference to the long-term clinical management at present.

It is, however, important, when setting up research studies into ME/CFS and Long Covid, to have sufficient patient numbers to allow sub-group analysis according to the type of onset, confirmed infection or not, duration, and type of symptoms. This requires clear and detailed initial histories.

FURTHER READING

Chu L, Valencia IJ, Garvert DW, Montoya JG. Onset patterns and course of myalgic encephalomyelitis/chronic fatigue syndrome. *Front Pediatr.* 2019;7:12. *htttps://doi.org/10.3389/fped.2019.00012.*

Vaes AW, Van Herck M, Deng Q, Delbressine JM, Jason LA, Spruit MA. Symptom-based clusters in people with ME/CFS: an illustration of clinical variety in a cross-sectional cohort. *J Transl Med.* 2023;21(1):112. *https://doi.org/10.1186/s12967-023-03946-6.*

4.7 Long Covid

Descriptions of 'Long Covid', a persistent fatigue syndrome indistinguishable from ME/CFS were noted from the earliest stages of the pandemic. None of the symptoms described in Long Covid were unknown to the descriptions provided by thousands of patients with ME/CFS over the years, apart from the very specific symptom of anosmia (see next). What was much more interesting was that, rather than being brushed off by the medical profession, these patients were taken much more seriously, in part because a significant number of early sufferers were from medical and nursing professions. This in turn led to much more intensive early investigation, which has been valuable in learning about how post-infectious fatigue develops.

In a study carried out by the Centres for Disease Control and Prevention in the USA, 18% of those surveyed said they experienced Long Covid. Likewise, a study by the Academic of Sciences in the USA demonstrated that recovery from Long Covid peaks around 6–12 months but that 18–22% of patients ill at 5 months are still ill at 12 months. This is a very similar pattern to that previously described in ME/CFS, where those who are going to make a recovery usually show evidence of this by 6–12 months and thereafter, the chances of improvement decline. Both Long Covid and ME/CFS show features of a relapsing remitting disease.

However, when looking at ME/CFS as a whole about 50% of patients give a clear history of an acute illness, usually viral-sounding. In almost all cases, no viral cause is ever identified, mainly because the critical point for accurate diagnostic tests has long passed or alternatively that we have been looking for signs of infection in the periphery when they are actually in the brain. Long Covid has been different, because of the universal use of acute testing for COVID-19 infection, which has enabled the persistent chronic fatigue after infection to be directly linked to a specific infection.

In the past, wherever there has been an identifiable infection preceding the onset of chronic fatigue it has been the custom to label this as post-infectious chronic fatigue, although this term up until now has rarely been clinically or therapeutically helpful, as, like a hit and run driver, the triggering infection has long since disappeared by the time of assessment, leaving the person with typical ME/CFS symptoms. Whether the current work on the persistence of COVID-19 and the potential links of ME/CFS to herpesviruses will change this approach remains to be seen. The use of new tests to identify viral persistence gives new possibilities to identify causative organisms with increased diagnostic certainty.

The fact that the acute illness with SARS CoV2 creates some symptoms such as anosmia, that are not seen in ME/CFS, has been used as an argument that the two conditions are distinct. However, this is not relevant as the anosmia is a very specific immediate effect of the viral infection. It appears that the olfactory cells in the nose are directly infected by the virus in the early stages, using the ACE2 receptor. Prolonged anosmia however, leads to chronic brain changes in the way smell is is perceived and this will be persistent and will therefore accompany Long Covid, although it is not part of the chronic fatigue response. This virus-specific effect does not have an impact on whether someone is likely to develop Long Covid. The anosmia may be persistent and studies have shown that this alone has a major detrimental effect on the mental health of patients with Long Covid. Rehabilitation therapy is available.

Comparative studies have confirmed the high degree of similarity between the Long Covid and ME/CFS (see Wong et al.). For the time being, Long Covid simply remains a subset of ME/CFS, where the triggering infection is known.

FURTHER READING

Annesley SJ, Missailidis D, Heng B, Josev EK, Armstrong CW. Unravelling shared mechanisms: insights from recent ME/CFS research to illuminate Long Covid pathologies. *Trends Mol Med.* 2024;**30**:443–8. *https://doi.org/10.1016/j.mol med.2024.02.003.*

Burges Watson DL, Campbell M, Hopkins C, et al. Altered smell and taste: anosmia, parosmia and the impact of long COVID-19. *PLoS ONE.* 2021;**16**(9):e0256998. *https:// doi.org/10.1371/journal.pone.0256998.*

Saniasiaya J, Narayanan P. Parosmia post COVID-19: an unpleasant manifestation of Long Covid syndrome. *Postgrad Med J.* 2022;**98**(e2):e96. *https://doi.org/10.1136/postgradm edj-2021-139855.*

Tsilingiris D, Vallianou NG, Karampela I, et al. Laboratory findings and biomarkers in Long Covid: what do we know so far? Insights into epidemiology, pathogenesis, therapeutic perspectives and challenges. *Int J Mol Sci.* 2023;**24**(13):10458. *https://doi.org/10.3390/ijms241310458.*

Turner S, Khan MA, Putrino D, Woodcock A, Kell DB, Pretorius E. Long Covid: pathophysiological factors and abnormalities of coagulation. *Trends Endocrinol Metab.* 2023;**34**(6):321–44. *https://doi.org/10.1016/j.tem.2023.03.002.*

Wong TL, Weitzer DJ. Long Covid and myalgic encephalomyelitis/chronic fatigue syndrome (ME/CFS)—a systemic review and comparison of clinical presentation and symptomatology. *Medicina.* 2021;**57**(5):418. *https://doi.org/10.3390/medicina5 7050418*

4.8 Fibromyalgia and chronic regional pain syndrome

4.8.1 Fibromyalgia

Fibromyalgia (FM) is a chronic condition characterized by muscular and joint pain with disability, where there is no evidence of active inflammatory arthritis or myositis. Symptoms include increased sensitivity to pain, muscle and joint stiffness, fatigue, brain fog ('fibro-fog'), headaches, and symptoms of IBS. The cause is unknown, although there is a potential link to HHV-6b infection, so this may put it into the same category as ME/CFS, where herpesviruses are also on the list of potential causes. It may occur after severe physical and/or emotional stress and may be seen in PTSD. It may be associated with temporomandibular joint disorder. The diagnosis is made clinically on the basis of the number of specific points on the body that are tender (>11/18 is considered diagnostic). Fatigue is a usual accompaniment, meaning that there is considerable overlap with ME/CFS. Equally, many patients with ME/CFS have typical fibromyalgia pain. Not all CFS patients have FM-like symptoms and there is a spectrum from none to quite severe. There is also an overlap of FM with complex regional pain syndromes (see next). Treatment of FM follows similar lines to ME/CFS, but there are specific guidelines available.

Recent studies using micro-RNA (MiRNA) detection have shown that it is possible to distinguish between FM, ME/CFS, and ME/CFS with FM. With the overlap in symptomatology of the two conditions this may become more important, although at the moment the tests are research only.

FURTHER READING

Macfarlane GJ, Kronisch C, Dean LE, et al. EULAR revised recommendations for the management of fibromyalgia. *Ann Rheum Dis.* 2017;**76**(2):318–28. *https://doi.org/10.1136/annrheumdis-2016-209724.*

Nepotchatykh E, Caraus I, Elremaly W, et al. Circulating micro-RNA expression signatures accurately discriminate myalgic encephalomyelitis from fibromyalgia and comorbid conditions. *Sci Rep.* 2023;**13**:1896. *https://doi.org/10.1038/s41598-023-28955-9.*

4.8.2 Complex regional pain syndrome (CRPS)

This is a condition, previously called Sudek's atrophy, reflex sympathetic dystrophy, causalgia, or algoneurodystrophy, with marked pain in limbs associated with marked vasomotor colour changes and sometimes muscle wasting. It is strongly associated with fibromyalgia and is more common in females. Two types are identified: CRPS-1 occurs when there is no nerve injury, while CRPS-2 is associated with specific nerve injury. There are links to PTSD and depression. No mechanism is yet known, but it has been suggested that the illness forms part of a spectrum of autoimmune dysautonomias. It is thought to be linked to abnormalities in the peripheral C-type pain fibres and the autonomic nervous system. As well as pain, there is often marked fatigue. Diagnostic criteria and management are discussed by Harden et al. (2022). Management is complex and usually requires referral to a specialist pain management service.

FURTHER READING

Harden RN, McCabe CS, Goebel A, et al. Complex regional pain syndrome: practical diagnostic and treatment guidelines. *Pain Med.* 2022;**23**(Suppl 1):S1–53. *https://doi.org/10.1093/pm/pnac046.*

Shoenfeld Y, Ryabkova VA, Scheibenbogen C, et al. Complex syndromes of chronic pain, fatigue and cognitive impairment linked to autoimmune dysautonomia and small fiber neuropathy. *Clin Immunol.* 2020;**214**:10838. *https://doi.org/10.1016/j.clim.2020.108384.*

4.9 Other conditions associated with ME/CFS and Long Covid

4.9.1 Positional orthostatic tachycardia syndrome (POTS)

This is an autonomic dysfunction syndrome that is strongly associated with chronic fatigue syndrome, although it may occur in the absence of fatigue. It is commoner in young patients and is characterized by an abnormal tachycardia on changing from lying to standing (either a rise of >30 bpm, or a rate >120 bpm). Symptoms may include postural dizziness and/or tachycardia. It is important to identify these patients as drug therapy will control the heart rate and improve symptoms. Patients with POTS as well as CFS will usually not notice dramatic improvements in their fatigue from therapy and referral to CFS/ME therapy teams is required for fatigue management. Diagnosis should be undertaken by a falls and syncope service with access to tilt table testing.

FURTHER READING

Hoad A, Spickett G, Elliott J, Newton J. Postural orthostatic tachycardia syndrome is an under-recognized condition in chronic fatigue syndrome. QJM: *Int J Med.* 2008;**101**;961–5. *https://doi.org/10.1093/qjmed/hcn123.*

4.9.2 Recurrent vasovagal syncope (young patients) with fatigue

This is the blood pressure equivalent of POTS and is also an autonomic dysfunction syndrome, but where there is marked and inappropriate postural hypotension, often associated with syncope. It is most commonly seen in children and young adults with ME/CFS. Diagnosis and management through a falls and syncope service with access to tilt table testing is required. Cerebral blood flow may be markedly reduced on even minor tilting, without blood pressure and heart rate changes. Drug therapy may improve the syncopal tendency but will not resolve the fatigue.

It is particularly important to identify postural autonomic syndromes as patients with these syndromes in association with chronic fatigue are more likely to become bed-bound, as getting up makes them feel much worse. Deconditioning and worsening of the postural symptoms then follow. Postural exercise training can be used to supplement drug therapy. Encouraging fluid intake, avoidance of caffeinated drinks, and increasing salt intake can be helpful.

FURTHER READING

van Campen CL, Rowe PC, Visser FC. Comparison of a 20 degree and 70 degree tilt test in adolescent myalgic encephalomyelitis/chronic fatigue syndrome (ME/CFS) patients. *Front Pediatr.* 2023;11:1169447. *https://doi.org/10.3389/fped.2023.1169447.*

4.9.3 DEMS with polyalgia

DEMS stands for dry eyes and mouth syndrome. These patients have features suggesting Sjögren's syndrome, with dry eyes and mouth, non-specific generalized aching, and debilitating fatigue. Blood tests show that, unlike true Sjögren's syndrome, these patients do not have elevated inflammatory markers, elevated immunoglobulins, or positive autoantibodies. Published evidence suggests that they should be managed as CFS/ME.

FURTHER READING

Mariette X, Caudmont C, Bergé E, Desmoulins F, Pinabel F. Dry eyes and mouth syndrome or sicca, asthenia and polyalgia syndrome?. *Rheumatology (Oxford).* 2003;**42**:914–15. *https://doi.org/10.1093/rheumatology/keg226.*

4.9.4 Reactive hypoglycaemia

Some patients with ME/CFS who follow unusual diets with inadequate carbohydrate content may develop secondary insulin oversensitivity, leading to late reactive hypoglycaemia 2–4 hours after carbohydrate intake, with symptoms of dizziness, faintness, nausea, and sweating. This often reinforces the impression that they are intolerant of carbohydrates, which they reduce still further, increasing the symptoms! The diagnosis is made by a four-hour glucose tolerance test, which will demonstrate late hypoglycaemia. Management is by regular small meals of complex carbohydrates, avoidance of refined sugars, and management of the ME/CFS in the usual way.

FURTHER READING

Bethune CA, Gompels MM, Spickett GP. Physiological effects of starvation interpreted as food allergy. *BMJ*. 1999;**319**(7205):304–5. *https://doi.org/10.1136/bmj.319.7205.304*.

Heuft L, Bravenboer B, Ziekenhuis C. Functional hypoglycaemia postulated as cause of chronic fatigue syndrome. *BMJ*. 1993;**307**(6906):735. *https://www.bmj.com/content/307/6906/735.1*.

4.9.5 Irritable bowel syndrome and irritable bladder syndrome (interstitial cystitis)

Almost all patients with ME/CFS have symptoms of IBS. If the patient has a prior diagnosis of IBS, the source of the diagnosis should be checked, including verification of the investigations carried out. Patients should be advised to follow the BDA/NICE guidance on dietary management of IBS. This may include trials of the FODMAP diet. Symptoms of nocturnal diarrhoea or blood in the stools suggest inflammatory bowel syndromes and require further investigation. CFS therapy intervention is not appropriate until such investigations have been completed and confirmed as normal. The baseline blood testing recommended by NICE includes a serological test for coeliac—this should be done early in the illness. A positive result is an indication for referral for endoscopy and duodenal biopsy.

A smaller proportion of patients with ME/CFS complain of irritable bladder syndrome, with frequency and dysuria. This may overlap with interstitial cystitis, which can cause bladder pain. Some patients' irritable bladder may be helped by dietary manipulation, although there is no convincing evidence that there is an allergic (IgE)-mediated cause for the condition.

It has been suggested that sympathetic dysfunction is the link between the bladder and bowel symptoms and chronic fatigue, although this is unlikely to be the only link.

FURTHER READING

Martínez-Martínez L-A, Mora T, Vargas A, et al. Sympathetic nervous system dysfunction in fibromyalgia, chronic fatigue syndrome, irritable bowel syndrome, and interstitial cystitis: a review of case-control studies. *J Clin Rheumatol*. 2014;**20**(3):146–50. *https://doi.org/10.1097/RHU.0000000000000089*.

4.9.6 Mast cells

There appears to be a possible link between excessive mast cell activation and ME/CFS. This may be due to the Th2-skewing of immune responses found in long-term cases of ME/CFS. MCAS is distinct from mastocytocytosis: there is no evidence of clinical proliferation of mast cells in MCAS and tryptase levels are usually not elevated. Mast cells release proinflammatory mediators and can interact with the autonomic nervous syndrome. The precise role that mast cells play in the generation of ME/CFS and Long Covid remains to be fully explored.

FURTHER READING

Theoharides TC, Twahir A, Kempuraj D. Mast cells in the autonomic nervous system and potential role in disorders with dysautonomia and neuroinflammation. *Ann Allergy Asthma Immunol.* 2024;132(4):440–54. *https://doi.org/10.1016/j.anai.2023.10.032.*

4.9.7 Migraine

There is quite a strong association between chronic migrainous headache and ME/CFS. The boundary between chronic migraine and ME/CFS is blurred and it is valuable to think about the condition if there is unusually severe or frequent headache, with visual disturbance in the context of fatigue and then seek an opinion from a neurologist interested in migraine, as there are new treatments available to manage chronic migraine. Chronic migraine, properly defined, is a cause of secondary chronic fatigue (refer to section 4.2).

4.9.8 Other possible causes of chronic fatigue

Over many years a range of other putative causes of chronic fatigue (ME/CFS) have been proposed. The evidence is weak. Included in this list are mercury (in dental amalgam), cadmium, and other heavy metals. While metals such as mercury and cadmium do cause medical syndromes on heavy exposure, these syndromes are distinct from ME/CFS. There is no convincing evidence associating mercury amalgam with an increased risk of ME/CFS, although if old filling are being replaced, it may be wise for white fillings to be used, as fresh fillings release higher amounts of mercury than old fillings.

Pesticides, including organophosphates, can cause very specific neurological syndromes, which often have chronic fatigue as an element (refer to section 4.5.17 earlier in this chapter). The at-risk population tends to be those working in agriculture or crop-spraying. Occupational history is, therefore, important. There is no good evidence to suggest that ME/CFS as a whole is related to these compounds.

CHAPTER 5

Theories of causation

KEY POINTS

- Many research studies into ME/CFS and Long Covid are hampered by insufficient numbers, lack of appropriate control groups, and inappropriate patient groups (longstanding and new patients combined).
- The exact pathways causing chronic fatigue and associated symptoms in ME/CFS and Long Covid have not yet been fully explored.
- Many different viruses and some bacteria may trigger chronic fatigue. In some cases of Long Covid, there is evidence for persistent viral presence in the brain, long after the acute infection has resolved. Further work is required to identify viral persistence in ME/CFS.
- A disordered immune response to infection is important. There are markers of chronic inflammation.
- Chronic viral persistence may lead to chronic inflammation, including neuroinflammation. This can lead to endocrine abnormalities due to interference with the HPA.
- Marked changes in brain structure and function have been identified in both ME/CFS and Long Covid. These include changes in the brainstem in areas controlling breathing.
- Abnormalities of mitochondrial function have been described.
- In the early stages of Long Covid, platelet and clotting disorders have been described. It is not known whether these are seen in the early phase of ME/CFS.
- There are possible links to the gut microbiome and diet.
- Genetic studies have not identified any clear pattern of predisposing genes, but HLA-DQ2 is associated with resistance to SARS-CoV2 infection.
- Psychiatric and psychological disorders are secondary to a primary post-infective chronic neuroinflammatory state, possibly associated with persistent viral infection of brain tissue.

5.1 Introduction to causation

For a condition that many have considered to be psychological or factitious, there is a remarkably large body of studies about causes. Many of these are small studies and up until now have mostly been inconclusive. In many cases studies have been undertaken from the perspective of proving that the illness isn't medical or is the same as depression, etc. Because so much of the research has been of poor quality, with inappropriate methodology and small numbers of patients, it has been impossible to draw firm conclusions. The poor quality of much past research, together with the perception that the illness is all in the mind, has also made it harder to get funding for proper studies.

There are a number of basic problems with any research into ME/CFS and Long Covid, which have been well-reviewed by Høeg et al. (2024). While these authors have focused on Long Covid, exactly the same constraints apply to research on ME/CFS. These can be characterized as: numbers, apples and pears, and phenomenology (primary versus secondary pathology). Other key issues are the presence of control groups (many studies lack any type of control group) and how well-matched the controls are.

5.1.1 Numbers

For a common condition, recruitment of adequate numbers of patients should be relatively easy. Usually, lack of funding has meant that studies are too small to produce meaningful (i.e. statistically significant) results. Recruitment difficulty has also meant that patients who might have different aetiologies or are at different stages of their illness are lumped together, which further dilutes any trends to significance. Where patient and control numbers are small, then the possibility of sampling bias exists, which will invalidate studies.

5.1.2 Apples and pears

Most people, including most non-specialist doctors, assume that ME/CFS and Long Covid are homogenous illnesses. As discussed in the previous chapter, ME/CFS covers a range of different presentations. Because these different presentations are never considered during recruitment to research studies and/or the numbers recruited are too small for meaningful sub-group analysis, apples end up being mixed with pears, and the end result is meaningless or misleading results. Many studies have included patients who have not been rigorously assessed for confounding medical or psychological problems by experienced physicians. The lack of any clear biomarker(s) for ME/CFS means that selection is difficult and dependent on diagnostic criteria which are not necessarily specific to ME/CFS.

Studies often also include newly diagnosed and longstanding patients. The biomarker signature in the two groups may be very different, but this itself has never been investigated, partly because, up until the onset of COVID-19, ME/CFS patients were never seen in the early acute phase of their illness, but only when they had been ill for a minimum of 4–6 months. Again, it is necessary to have sufficient numbers to be able to separate the relatively acute from the very chronic patients and analyse them separately. Only if the two groups have the same biomarker profile is it justified to combine the groups.

Long Covid, however, is much easier to study as there are clear biomarkers for the infection with an identifiable time point for infection, which then makes large-scale studies feasible and practical. The result is that much of what we know about the acute-onset pathology of ME/CFS is currently being extrapolated from studies on Long Covid. However, similar constraints apply concerning the appropriateness of research methodology. Research confirms that the immune abnormalities and other neurological and biochemical changes evolve during the course of the illness, which makes it even more important to select patients for studies at the same stage of their illness.

5.1.3 Phenomenology

Working out what is cause and what is effect in ME/CFS is hugely difficult. Because the previous diagnostic criteria for ME/CFS in the UK required the illness to have been present for at least 4 months before referral to specialist services can be actioned, researchers in such specialized units have missed the most interesting phase of the illness, i.e. the initiation phase. The latest guidance now specifies 6 weeks, before referral, but there will then be a further gap until the patient is actually seen! It then becomes hard to determine whether a particular set of biological findings are directly related to or are the cause of ME/CFS, or are changes that have occurred as a consequence of ME/CFS. Measuring abnormalities in IgG subclasses in a small group of patients with ME/CFS, as I did in the early 1990s, and showing that they diverge from the expected normal ranges in healthy adults really does not advance our understanding of the cause of ME/CFS. It is merely a phenomenon of uncertain significance. There are many similar studies!

Point studies (studies taken once at a single point in the patient's illness) are particularly likely to fall into this category. In most cases of ME/CFS there will not be any pre-illness samples that can be studied, so an individual patient's pre-illness baseline is unknown. In the case of the IgG subclass study, it may be that the abnormalities that we found were actually present before the illness began and are actually normal for that patient. Alternatively, it may be that, while present beforehand, they represented a particular risk factor for developing the illness. Finally, it may be that they have developed as a result of the illness. None of these three possibilities could be answered in the study, rendering it simply a measurement of a phenomenon at a single point in the patient's life story.

Interpretation of the significance of abnormal findings in patients with ME/CFS is therefore fraught with difficulty. All research studies need to be analysed with these considerations in mind.

Although the evidence is now turning against ME/CFS being a psychiatric or psychological disease, there is no doubt from research studies that the psychosocial background plays an important role as a co-factor in the onset and perpetuation of the disease. ME/CFS is more likely to develop in people who have had a major stressful life event in the year preceding the onset. This can include divorce, bereavement, and unemployment. The major flooding in Cumbria that occurred on two occasions during my working career led a to a spike in cases of ME/CFS among those worst affected by the floods. Studies have also shown that people who develop ME/CFS are more likely to have a past history of abuse, which may be physical, mental, or sexual. In many cases, patients do not volunteer this information unless specifically asked. As we know that any sort of severe acute or chronic stress has a major impact on immune function which in turn predisposes to infection, it becomes easier to see the chain of events that culminates in ME/CFS. There is abundant evidence that stress has a major impact on immune function, with increased susceptibility to infection. During the pandemic, health and social care staff were stressed to the extreme, making it more likely that they would develop COVID-19 and, in turn, would be more likely to develop Long Covid as a result.

Simplistic models of a single event (infection) causing ME/CFS are most likely wrong. As will be discussed, a multistep process is much more likely. Chronic fatigue may actually be the end result of this series of steps, not the beginning of the illness. As well as a predisposing psychological (stress-related) background, there may be subtle abnormalities in the immune system, either pre-existing, triggered by stress or changes caused by a triggering infection. Whether there is a genetic predisposition is also still unclear.

The science of both ME/CFS and Long Covid are now converging, with more clinical scientists recognizing the overwhelming similarities in symptomatology and biology between the two illnesses and are now attempting a synthesis of the science generated separately for the two conditions. See, for example: Annesley et al. (2024), Tate et al. (2023), Komaroff & Lipkin (2021), and Komaroff & Lipkin (2023). These papers provide very succinct reviews of our current understanding of the pathology of both ME/CFS and Long Covid and discuss the convergence of the science.

A great problem for both conditions is the absence of a simple biomarker that positively identifies the conditions with a high degree of sensitivity and specificity. Many attempts have been made over the years, using increasingly complicated screens of biomarkers, over 40 in some studies, to identify a unique and diagnostic pattern. These have failed, leaving diagnosis still rooted in clinical assessment, based on symptom patterns and the absence of any potential confounding diagnoses. The application of machine learning to studies of multiple biomarkers is making it more likely that we will be able to pick out markers which give useful information on the diseases.

For many of the conditions outlined in Chapter 4.2, the mechanism of fatigue is unknown, or indeed ignored! Hopefully, the current wave of investigation will identify whether the fatigue of all chronic conditions has the same physiological basis.

FURTHER READING

Annesley SJ, Missailidis D, Heng B, Josev EK, Armstrong CW. Unravelling shared mechanisms: insights from recent ME/CFS research to illuminate Long Covid pathologies. *Trends Mol Med.* 2024;**30**(5):443–58. *https://doi.org/10.1016/j.molmed.2024.02.003.*

Deumer US, Varesi A, Floris V, et al. Myalgic encephalomyelitis/chronic fatigue syndrome (ME/CFS): an overview. *J Clin Med.* 2021;**10**(20):4786. *https://doi.org/10.3390/jcm1 0204786.*

CHAPTER 5

Høeg TB, Ladhani S, Prasad V. How methodological pitfalls have created widespread misunderstanding about Long Covid. *BMJ Evid Based Med.* 2024;29(3):142–6. *https://doi.org/10.1136/bmjebm-2023-112338.*

Komaroff AL, Lipkin WI. Insights from myalgic encephalomyelitis/chronic fatigue syndrome may help unravel the pathogenesis of postacute COVID-19 syndrome. *Trends Mol Med.* 2021;27(9):895–906. *https://doi.org/10.1016/j.molmed.2021.06.002.*

Komaroff AL, Lipkin WI. ME/CFS and Long Covid share similar symptoms and biological abnormalities: road map to the literature. *Front Med.* 2023;10:1187163. *https://doi.org/10.3389/fmed.2023.1187163.*

Li J, Zhou Y, Ma J, et al. The long-term health outcomes, pathophysiological mechanisms and multidisciplinary management of Long Covid. *Sig Transduct Target Ther.* 2023;8:416. *https://doi.org/10.1038/s41392-023-01640-z.*

Nacul L, O'Boyle S, Palla L, et al. How myalgic encephalomyelitis/chronic fatigue syndrome (ME/CFS) progresses: the natural history of ME/CFS. *Front Neurol.* 2020;11:826. *https://doi.org/10.3389/fneur.2020.00826.*

Tate WP, Walker MOM, Peppercorn K, Blair ALH, Edgar CD. Towards a better understanding of the complexities of myalgic encephalomyelitis/chronic fatigue syndrome and Long Covid. *Int J Mol Sci.* 2023; 24(6):5124. *https://doi.org/10.3390/ijms24065124.*

5.2 Genetics

ME/CFS over the last 50 years appears to be a sporadic illness, although as discussed in Chapter 1, in the past it has been strongly associated with apparent epidemics. While there are occasional families where more than one family member is affected, concrete evidence of heritability is absent. Where mothers and children are affected, some have postulated that the children 'learn' illness behaviour from the parent. While this is possible, it also remains possible that there is a genetic link in at least some cases.

The possibility that both ME/CFS and Long Covid represent an autoimmune disease of the brain, triggered by infection also provides a possible genetic background as almost all autoimmune diseases are linked to a particular autoimmune genetic phenotype. Autoimmune diseases in general tend to be more common in females than in males and, in some cases (e.g. systemic lupus erythematous), the skewing towards females is quite extreme (10:1). In ME/CFS, the female to male ratio is around 3:1. Similar findings have been established in Long Covid.

So far genetic studies have not confirmed that ME/CFS or Long Covid are related to abnormalities of single genes, except in Long Covid where there have been close family members who have had unusually severe COVID-19 infection and abnormalities in the X-linked gene for TLR7 have been identified, which would impair both Type I and Type II interferon responses to infection. Other abnormalities of immune function genes, such as *MBL* and Pentraxin 3, may also contribute to COVID-19 susceptibility. The *ACE* gene has been implicated in COVID-19, as it codes for a protein that the virus uses to enter cells. Large studies on ME/CFS have identified 333 genes with an association with ME/CFS, including a number with an impact on immune function, including HLA antigens (HLA-A, HLA-C, HLA-DQA1, HLA-DRB1), Tyk2, Toll-like receptors, and genes controlling mast cells and microglia, and brain function, including HPA function, surface receptors, and ion channels (thus impairing intercellular signalling).

A challenge study (Lindeboom et al., 2024) to deliberately infect volunteers with a low dose of the original SARS-CoV2 nasally under controlled conditions identified that the volunteers could be divided into three groups: those who developed a sustained infection with multiple positive tests and cold-like symptoms, those who developed a transient infection with single or intermittent positive tests and few symptoms and a third group with no positive tests and no symptoms. Group 2 had a rapid accumulation of immune cells in the nose within 24 hours, whereas in Group 1 the immune response did not start until 5 days, allowing infection to be established. High expression of HLA-DQ2 prior to infection was strongly associated with preventing sustained infection. It has long been known that, when studying infectious diseases, there are always populations, usually small, who do not develop infection despite exposure.

So far genome-wide association studies (GWAS) have not identified any reproducible patterns in studies on cohorts of patients with ME/CFS, despite five studies, using ME/CFS patients in the UK Biobank. However, it may be that the number of cases in the Biobank is too low for accurate assessment and a much larger study of robustly diagnosed case may be more helpful. Recruitment to a much larger study, DecodeME, is now underway.[1] In Long Covid, GWAS has identified FOXP4 as a risk factor for developing the condition, but this gene may also be a risk factor for severe COVID-19 infection in the first place and severe infection itself is a risk factor for Long Covid.

Since it is highly probable that ME/CFS is caused by a wide range of different pathogens, the susceptibility genes may be different, depending on which type of infection is the trigger. This may explain why previous attempts to isolate a genetic predisposition to ME/CFS have failed. Only when we are able to conclusively link every case of ME/CFS to a particular infective trigger and then analyse the genetics for each infection will we begin to see patterns emerging.

FURTHER READING

Devereux-Cooke A, Leary S, McGrath SJ, et al. DecodeME: community recruitment for a large genetics study of myalgic encephalomyelitis/chronic fatigue syndrome. *BMC Neurol*. 2022;22(1):269. *https://doi.org/10.1186/s12883-022-02763-6*.

Dibble JJ, McGrath SJ, Ponting CP. Genetic risk factors of ME/CFS: a critical review. *Hum Mol Genet*. 2020;29(R1):R117–24. *https://doi.org/10.1093/hmg/ddaa169*.

Lammi V, Nakanishi T, Jones SE, et al. Genome-wide association study of Long Covid. *medRxiv*. 2023:2023–6. *https://doi.org/10.1101/2023.06.29.23292056*.

---

[1] See DecodeMe, *https://www.decodeme.org.uk*

Lindeboom RG, Worlock KB, Dratva LM, et al. Human SARS-CoV-2 challenge uncovers local and systemic response dynamics. *Nature*. 2024;**631**(8019):189–98. *https://doi.org/10.1038/s41586-024-07575-x*.

Lv Y, Zhang T, Cai J, Huang C, Zhan S, Liu J. Bioinformatics and systems biology approach to identify the pathogenetic link of Long Covid and myalgic encephalomyelitis/chronic fatigue syndrome. *Front Immunol*. 2022;**13**:952987. *https://doi.org/10.3389/fimmu.2022.952987*.

Sylvester SV, Rusu R, Chan B, Bellows M, O'Keefe C, Nicholson S. Sex differences in sequelae from COVID-19 infection and in Long Covid syndrome: a review. *Curr Med Res Opin*. 2022;**38**(8):1391–9. *https://doi.org/10.1080/03007995.2022.2081454*.

Tziastoudi M, Cholevas C, Stefanidis I, Theoharides TC. Genetics of COVID-19 and myalgic encephalomyelitis/chronic fatigue syndrome: a systematic review. *Ann Clin Transl Neurol*. 2022;**9**(11):1838–57. *https://doi.org/10.1002/acn3.51631*.

5.3 Infection

The history of ME/CFS is full of attempts to link the disease to a specific infection and for reasons already discussed, this is unhelpful (see Chapter 1). Almost all infections are accompanied acutely by fatigue, this being part of the body's normal response to infection. As there are, as yet, no robust predictive markers for those who will go on to develop chronic fatigue, i.e. those whose acute fatigue does not resolve, it is difficult to identify those for whom infection screening may be helpful, unless there are some specific indicators or the acute infection is part of an epidemic such as influenza or coronavirus, where testing is mandated. It may be that the markers of risk will vary according to the nature of the initiating infection. As discussed next, some specific risk factors for developing Long Covid are beginning to emerge.

In the majority of cases the diagnosis of ME/CFS cannot be considered until a period of time has passed (usually at least 6 weeks, but often longer), which means that by the time the diagnosis is considered it is too late to do any antigen/DNA/RNA tests for infection. In most cases, any active infection has long since disappeared. Occasionally antibody tests may be helpful, but only where the test is for an unusual infection. The difficulties of testing for Epstein–Barr virus (EBV) as a cause have been alluded to already, as the infection is so common that 95% of adults will have evidence of previous infection. In most cases any putative causative infection has long since gone, like a hit-and-run incident, where there are long-term injuries consequent on a single point of injury. It is also highly likely that many different infections can result in ME/CFS, depending on individual susceptibility and therefore it is equally unlikely that there will be a single causative infection.

Attempts have been made over the years to attribute ME/CFS to chronic infection, but none of the studies so far have stood up to rigorous testing. Where there is evidence of chronic infection, then that clearly indicates an attributable cause for the fatigue and should, if appropriate, receive relevant treatment.

Usually, but not always, appropriate treatment will resolve or at least improve the fatigue. There will usually be pointers to risks for chronic infections, such as brucellosis, toxoplasmosis, Lyme disease (borreliosis), tuberculosis, and HIV.

In the middle of the 20th century before the widespread introduction of polio vaccines, abortive poliovirus infection was considered as a possibility, particularly in association with the epidemic form of ME/CFS. In the 1960s, there was a lot of focus on EBV as a trigger, although as discussed earlier, this was largely driven by the benefits system in the USA, which required patients with ME/CFS to have evidence of EBV infection before they could claim benefits. There is no doubt that severe cases of confirmed acute EBV infection can trigger subsequent ME/CFS, but there is no current evidence that EBV is a cause of the majority of cases of ME/CFS.

In the 1980s and 1990s, there was interest in the role of coxsackieviruses and other enteroviruses as aetiological agents in ME/CFS. Poliovirus is a member of the Enterovirus family, so this potentially linked with earlier studies on the epidemic forms of ME/CFS. This was largely based around a test for the common VP1 antigen. While the initial test was eventually discredited, interest in this class of viruses persisted. The introduction of the drug rintatolimod (Ampligen), a mismatched ds-DNA poly-inosine/cytosine), as an antiviral and immune stimulant which activates TLR3, has increased interest. Coronaviruses and enteroviruses share a number of similarities and both are single-stranded RNA viruses, although coronaviruses are enveloped but enteroviruses are not. They do however share very similar proteases. While COVID-19 (a coronavirus) can clearly cause an ME/CFS-like illness (Long Covid), the evidence for other enteroviruses remains circumstantial. As noted earlier in the history of ME/CFS (Chapter 1), the encephalitis lethargica pandemic has been linked possibly to human enterovirus infection. There has, therefore, been an upsurge of interest again in the potential role of enteroviruses in ME/CFS (O'Neal & Hanson, 2021 and Hanson, 2023).

In 2009 there was great excitement following the publication of a paper from the USA linking ME/CFS to infection with a murine retrovirus called XMRV. Clinics were inundated with requests from patients to be tested for this new virus. Sadly, other laboratories were unable to confirm this finding and, in the end, the original laboratory identified that there was cross-contamination of their cultures with the murine virus.

Most recently, there has been an upsurge in interest in the role human betaherpes virus 6 (HHV-6B) as a possible cause. This illness usually causes a mild disease, but like all herpesviruses, has the potential to remain dormant in the body after infection, kept under control by the immune response generated by the initial infection. Studies (on small numbers of patients) have shown that patients with ME/CFS had higher levels of HHV-6B and a related virus HHV-7, with levels of the virus in the blood being highest when symptoms were most severe. Increased levels of the virus may trigger flares, explaining why levels are highest when symptoms are most severe. It may be that reactivation is localized rather than generalized as post-mortem studies in patients with ME/CFS showed localization of HHV-6 activity to the brain and spinal cord. This was not found in patients who had died but had no evidence for ME/CFS. It may still be that the reappearance of the herpesviruses at intervals in patients with ME/CFS is still secondary to the flares of the ME/CFS caused by other triggers, rather than the virus being the trigger for the flares: a classic chicken-and-egg question that is very difficult to answer.

Triggering reactivation of HHV-6B, or other herpesviruses, may require another acute infection, for example COVID-19 or SARS (another coronavirus infection). We know that herpes simplex virus (HSV, the cause of cold sores) and shingles (chickenpox (varicella) virus) reactivate in the infected nerves when a person who has previously been infected with HSV or Varicella virus becomes unwell for any reason (e.g. another infection, severe stress). It is thought that the immune system's ability to control these latent viruses is impaired by other events, allowing the viruses to escape from suppression. The immune system may simply be distracted by fighting a different infection or the new event may simply suppress the immune system. We know that stress is a potent suppressor of the immune system.

Q-fever, due to Coxiella infection, has also been associated with a prolonged chronic fatigue. While prolonged doxycycline treatment may help and in most cases the fatigue resolves after 6 months in some cases the fatigue may be long term. Studies of this syndrome have shown similarities with ME/CFS. Q-fever is an unusual infection and tends to be confined to those with specific occupational risk factors. The association with an ME/CFS like illness does however reinforce the point that non-viral infections may also lead to an ME/CFS like illness, even after successful antibiotic therapy.

The concept that ME/CFS is linked to candida overgrowth and therefore that anti-candida diets are advisable and patients should be treated with anti-candida agents is a longstanding one, for which evidence is limited. Anti-candida diets avoid sugars and are 'healthy' and will reduce irritable bowel symptoms (see Chapter 8.13). There have been published reports to the effect that ME/CFS have higher levels of anti-candida antibodies in their blood, although this is not proof of causation.

A very interesting long-term study of the links between infection and the development of ME/CFS in Taiwan has been published (Chang et al., 2023). 395,811 patients with infection were studied over a 17-year period, together with controls. ME/CFS was more likely to develop in patients infected with *Mycobacterium tuberculosis*, *E. coli*, Varicella zoster virus, Candida, salmonella, *Staphylococcus aureus*, and influenza virus. Patients treated with antibiotics (doxycycline, azithromycin, moxifloxacin, levofloxacin, or ciprofloxacin) had a lower risk of developing ME/CFS. While this study does not confirm causation, it does suggest a link between ME/CFS and a range of potential infective agents.

The most dramatic and proven link of chronic fatigue with infection has occurred as a result of the SARS-CoV2 pandemic, where large numbers (millions) of people have developed long-lasting chronic fatigue with other typical ME/CFS features, with additional specific features unique to COVID-19-induced chronic fatigue such as persistent anosmia, for which there is a very clear reason, related to the effect of the virus on the nerves involved in smell. Prolonged fatigue of a similar nature was also reported after SARS infection (Long SARS). Studies on Long Covid have shown, contrary to expectations, there is evidence for viral persistence, with detection of spike and other viral proteins in between 30–60% of patients with Long Covid. Persistent production of viral proteins would certainly contribute to ongoing immune activation and chronic inflammation, with secondary impacts on multiple biological systems. If this is the process in Long Covid, then it begs the question if something similar is going on in ME/CFS and we just haven't been looking for the correct infection(s) or looking in the right place (brain, cerebrospinal fluid?).

The obvious role of SARS CoV2 in generating chronic fatigue has at last led to large-scale studies looking at the potential role of other common viruses in triggering chronic fatigue. The Covidence study in the UK has confirmed that other respiratory viruses, including the common cold, can cause similar long-term symptoms, with the severity and duration linked to the severity of the initial infection. The media have of course dubbed this 'Long Cold'! This adds weight to the view that chronic fatigue syndrome is likely to be a common sequela to many common infections and indicates that more extensive work is required to identify the underlying reasons why some people develop chronic fatigue and others don't and whether it is the same risk factors for every infection or whether the risk factors are unique to each infecting agent. It is also critical to understand whether patients labelled as ME/CFS have any evidence of persisting infection and this may require a re-think of how and where in the body persistence is sought.

When the data is collected, there are a large number of infections that are associated with 'unexplained post-acute infections syndromes', most of which are characterized by fatigue among other symptoms (Choutka et al 2022). While most are viral, including a range of tropical infections such as Ebola, dengue, other infections are also identified, such as a cause, such as Giardiasis, Q-fever, Lyme disease, and other tropical infections. Interestingly, in the light of the evidence of viral persistence in Long Covid, similar findings of viral persistence have been found with other viral infections causing prolonged symptoms, such as Ebola and West Nile virus infection.

There has been a lot of attention given to the theory that ME/CFS is due to chronic active Lyme disease, based on a number of unvalidated tests available privately. There is however no robust evidence to support this theory and the corollary that patients with ME/CFS should receive a long course of antibiotic therapy directed against this organism. However, like all acute infections, ME/CFS may result even after successful treatment of the acute infection, but there is no evidence so far that this is connected with bacterial persistence and a post-treatment Lyme disease syndrome is also recognized.

The development of ME/CFS may require multiple sequential events. It may be that individuals inherit an increased susceptibility to develop the illness (see earlier). Infection with a relatively harmless but persistent virus infection may then predispose to a more severe reactivation triggered by events later in life (stress, other infections). Finally, it may be that the second infection and the reactivation together predispose to the development of an abnormal immunological reaction (an autoimmune response).

It is not appropriate to make a diagnosis of ME/CFS in a person who has an identified active chronic infection until that person has received successful anti-infective treatment, if available. However, because any infection can be a trigger for ME/CFS, all of the chronic infections listed here may, even if successfully treated leave the person with a long-term ME/CFS, even when there are no obvious signs of active or chronic infection still present, although viral persistence needs to be considered.

As more and more viruses are associated with persistent fatigue, it has become clear that patients with Long Covid may experience an increase in symptoms as a result of other common viral infections such as the common cold. This parallels the situation that ME/CFS sufferers have long recognized: intercurrent infections always make their ME/CFS worse. This may be due to the reactivation of an original causative viral infection or due to secondary reactivation of the abnormal immune response.

There has been debate about whether COVID-19 vaccination is protective against the development of Long Covid. Several studies have suggested that Long Covid is more likely in the unvaccinated and that vaccination of up to two doses after the first infection may reduce symptoms of Long Covid, with the greatest benefit seen with mRNA vaccines. Against this are rare reports of vaccines triggering COVID-19-like symptoms and other autoimmune phenomena.

FURTHER READING

Ariza ME. Myalgic encephalomyelitis/chronic fatigue syndrome: the human herpesviruses are back! Biomolecules. 2021;11(2):185. *https://doi.org/10.3390/biom11020185.*

Bai NA, Richardson CS. Posttreatment Lyme disease syndrome and myalgic encephalomyelitis/chronic fatigue syndrome: a systematic review and comparison of pathogenesis. *Chronic Dis Transl Med.* 2023;9(3):183–90. *https://doi.org/10.1002/cdt3.74.*

Ceban F, Kulzhabayeva D, Rodrigues NB, et al. COVID-19 vaccination for the prevention and treatment of Long Covid: a systematic review and meta-analysis. *Brain Behav Immun.* 2023;111:211–29. *https://doi.org/10.1016/j.bbi.2023.03.022.*

Chang H, Kuo CF, Yu TS, Ke LY, Hung CL, Tsai SY. Increased risk of chronic fatigue syndrome following infection: a 17-year population-based cohort study. *J Transl Med.* 2023;21(1):804. *https://doi.org/10.1186/s12967-023-04636-z.*

Chen B, Julg B, Mohandas S, Bradfute SB. Viral persistence, reactivation, and mechanisms of Long Covid. *Elife.* 2023;12:e86015. *https://doi.org/10.7554/eLife.86015.*

Choutka J, Jansari V, Hornig M, Iwasaki A. Unexplained post-acute infection syndromes. *Nat Med.* 2022 May;28(5):911–23. *https://doi.org/10.1038/s41591-022-01810-6.*

Couzin-Frankel J, Vogel G. Vaccines may cause rare, Long Covid-like symptoms. *Science*. 2022;**375**(6579):364–6. *https://www.science.org/doi/pdf/10.1126/science.ada0536*.

Hanson MR. The viral origin of myalgic encephalomyelitis/chronic fatigue syndrome. *PLoS Pathog*. 2023;19(8):e1011523. *https://doi.org/10.1371/journal.ppat.1011523*.

Morroy G, Keijmel SP, Delsing CE, et al. Fatigue following acute Q-fever: a systematic literature review. *PLoS ONE*. 2016;11(5):e0155884. *https://doi.org/10.1371/journal. pone.0155884*.

Mozhgani SH, Rajabi F, Qurbani M, et al. Human herpesvirus 6 infection and risk of chronic fatigue syndrome: a systematic review and meta-analysis. *Intervirology*. 2022;**65**(1):49–57. *https://doi.org/10.1159/000517930*.

O'Neal AJ, Hanson MR. The enterovirus theory of disease etiology in myalgic encephalomyelitis/chronic fatigue syndrome: a critical review. *Front Med*. 2021;8:688486. *https://doi.org/10.3389/fmed.2021.688486*.

Proal AD, VanElzakker MB, Aleman S, et al. SARS-CoV-2 reservoir in post-acute sequelae of COVID-19 (PASC). *Nat Immunol*. 2023;24:1616–27. *https://doi.org/10.1038/s41 590-023-01601-2*.

Raijmakers RPH, Roerink ME, Jansen AFM, et al. Multi-omics examination of Q-fever fatigue syndrome identifies similarities with chronic fatigue syndrome. *J Transl Med*. 2020;18:448. *https://doi.org/10.1186/s12967-020-02585-5*.

Rasa S, Nora-Krukle Z, Henning N, et al. Chronic viral infections in myalgic encephalomyelitis/chronic fatigue syndrome (ME/CFS). *J Transl Med*. 2018;16:268. *https://doi.org/10.1186/s12967-018-1644-y*.

Salari N, Khodayari Y, Hosseinian-Far A, et al. Global prevalence of chronic fatigue syndrome among long COVID-19 patients: a systematic review and meta-analysis. *Biopsychosoc Med*. 2022;16(1):21. *https://doi.org/10.1186/s13030-022-00250-5*.

Sandler CX, Cvejic E, Valencia BM, Li H, Hickie IB, Lloyd AR. Predictors of chronic fatigue syndrome and mood disturbance after acute infection. *Front Neurol*. 2022;13:935442. *https://doi.org/10.3389/fneur.2022.935442*.

Strain WD, Sherwood O, Banerjee A, Van der Togt V, Hishmeh L, Rossman J. The impact of COVID vaccination on symptoms of Long Covid: an international survey of people with lived experience of Long Covid. *Vaccines*. 2022;10(5):652. *https://doi.org/10.3390/ vaccines10050652*.

Vivaldi G, Pfeffer PE, Talaei M et al. Long-term symptoms after COVID-19 vs. other acute respiratory infections: an analysis of data from the COVIDENCE UK study. *EClinicalMedicine*. 2023;65:102251.*https://doi.org/10.1016/j.eclinm.2023.102251*.

Wong TL, Weitzer DJ. Long Covid and myalgic encephalomyelitis/chronic fatigue syndrome (ME/CFS)—a systemic review and comparison of clinical presentation and symptomatology. *Medicina*. 2021;**57**(5):418. *https://doi.org/10.3390/medicina57050418*.

5.4 Brain abnormalities

Since COVID-19, there has been an increasing research interest in what is happening in the brain, both during acute infection and in Long Covid, which is now beginning to give significant insights into what physiologically constitutes fatigue and impacts on our understanding of ME/CFS.

MRI and functional MRI scans will usually be abnormal in both ME/CFS and Long Covid. Brainstem volume reductions have been reported in both ME/CFS and Long Covid. In Long Covid, reductions in brain volume and loss of both white and grey matter have been reported and appear to be associated with the severity of cognitive dysfunction, although not all studies have confirmed this. Reduced cerebral blood flow has been reported in both ME/CFS and Long Covid, leading to cerebral hypoperfusion. In particular, cerebral blood has been reported to drop in ME/CFS patients when they sit up and after walking, undoubtedly contributing to the worsening symptoms associated with posture and exercise. Positron emission tomography (PET) scanning confirms hypometabolism in the brains of ME/CFS and Long Covid patients. Both groups have abnormalities in the brain end of the HPA axis. It has been hypothesized that there is a defect in neurovascular coupling (the linkage of blood flow to active brain areas), leading to localized areas of poor perfusion and cerebral hypoxia. It has been suggested that peripherally produced inflammatory compounds generated in hypoxic muscles, such as bradykinin and heat-shock proteins, may exacerbate or cause this tendency, although the known autonomic dysregulation and ventricular dysfunction may equally well be the cause. Functional studies have shown abnormalities of the serotonin transporter system, which is likely to contribute to the depression experienced in ME/CFS. 5-HT hyperactivation has been proposed and investigated in a mouse model of fatigue.

There are pointers towards autoimmune damage in the brain, through auto-antibodies to beta-adrenergic and acetylcholine receptors (see section 5.5). In COVID-19 infection, acute brain involvement has been associated with intracerebral vascular injury, with microthrombi and the appearance in some cases of anti-phospholipid antibodies. Platelet function may be abnormal. The latter has not been particularly associated with ME/CFS, but then this group of patients are rarely seen in the initiation phase of the illness, so these changes may be missed. Other features of the anti-phospholipid syndrome are not seen in ME/CFS.

More recently, it has been proposed that there is chronic but fluctuating neuroinflammation linked to disordered function of the microglia and disruption of the normal blood–brain barrier function in ME/CFS and Long Covid. Microglia have a very important role in the maintenance of neuronal function and are involved in the maintenance and repair of synapses. This process is controlled by the presence of C1q on synapses. Abnormal microglial function is involved in neurodegenerative diseases such as Alzheimer's. The hypothesis of microglial involvement in the pathogenesis of ME/CFS and Long Covid has been proposed, and the evidence reviewed in two papers by Tate and colleagues in 2002 and 2023. It has been suggested that cytokines released by alveolar macrophages during the acute phase of SARS CoV2 infection of the lung may directly alter microglial function. Equally, the noted disorder of the complement system (see section 5.8) may also contribute to abnormal microglial function and subsequent neuroinflammation and damage to the normal maintenance of neuronal synapses.

A study from the University of Cambridge published in 2024 by Rua et al. (2024), using 7T-MRI demonstrated persistent abnormalities in the brainstem of patients with Long Covid, consistent with neuroinflammation and affecting particular areas controlling breathing. These important findings add to the evidence of Long Covid as a neuroinflammatory disease and suggest that the persistent breathing problems in Long Covid have a central mechanism. The air hunger described by patients with ME/CFS is likely to have the same underlying mechanism, although this remains to be confirmed. The clear evidence for brainstem involvement undoubtedly explains many of the autonomic problems seen in ME/CFS and Long Covid.

It is suggested that there may be damage, particularly to the paraventricular nucleus of the hypothalamus, which might interfere with normal stress responses and amplify 'danger' signals. Changes in the gut microbiome may affect this as well. This proposal would help link the diverse problems found in ME/CFS and Long Covid, such as disturbances of the HPA axis with hormonal abnormalities and serotoninergic pathways. This in turn links to the kynureine pathway of tryptophan metabolism. It has been suggested that elevated levels of serotonin may result from raised tryptophan levels, although this does not necessarily match with other data looking at the bowel.

Acute SARS-CoV2 and Long Covid and more recently ME/CFS have all been associated with disturbed clotting and the presence of micro thrombi, which potentially may be significant contributors to cerebral damage (see section 5.9). It has been proposed that there are abnormalities of the activation of microglia, which contribute to the neuroinflammation

Spinal cord fluid analysis (mass spectrometry, liquid chromatography, and peptide sequencing) has confirmed evidence of the presence of proteins associated with chronic inflammation and repair.

A recent large study has confirmed significant and apparently long-lasting problems with cognition and memory after COVID-19. A group at Imperial College, reporting in the New England Journal of Medicine, had started a study before the pandemic to look at how lifestyle affected cognition, measuring IQ. However, as COVID-19 became established, it became apparent that those who had severe COVID-19 (needing intensive care) or prolonged symptoms had a statistically significant and persistent reduction in IQ. The effect was still apparent a year after infection. They were also able to confirm that those who complained of 'brain fog' actually did have reductions in cognitive function. The effect appeared to be worse with the original strains but only marginal with the omicron variant. Vaccination appeared to be protective. The weakness of the study was of course that patients were not studied before and after. Notwithstanding, this study confirms that brain fog post-COVID-19 infection (Long Covid) is a real and measurable phenomenon. Of course, the next stage is to confirm that the same pattern is seen in ME/CFS, and perhaps after other severe infections. A similar effect has been seen in influenza infection, but the effect in COVID-19 is much larger. A similarly large study in Oslo confirmed memory impairment post-COVID-19.

At an entirely experimental level, luteolin a natural flavonoid which inhibits microglia or the synthetic tetramethoxyluteolin have been found to prevents neuoroinflammation and reduces cognitive dysfunction. This suggests that focus on the potential neuroinflammation in ME/CFS and Long Covid may lead to novel therapeutic agents. Low dose naltrexone, which has been suggested as a treatment for both ME/CFS and Long Covid has been shown to regulate microglia and reduce neuroinflammation. It modulates the expression of transient receptor potential melastain (TRPM3, a pain mediating receptor) in NK cells.

FURTHER READING

Almulla AF, Thipakorn Y, Zhou B, Vojdani A, Maes M. Immune activation and immune-associated neurotoxicity in Long Covid: a systematic review and meta-analysis of 103 studies comprising 58 cytokines/chemokines/growth factors. *Brain Behav Immun.* 2024;**122**:75–94. *https://doi.org/10.1016/j.bbi.2024.07.036.*

Ellingjord-Dale M, Brunvoll SH, Søraas A. Prospective memory assessment before and after COVID-19. *N Engl J Med.* 2024;**390**(9):863–5. *https://doi.org/10.1056/NEJMc 2311200.*

Hampshire A, Azor A, Atchison C, et al. Cognition and memory after COVID-19 in a large community sample. *N Engl J Med.* 2024;**390**(9):806–18. *https://doi.org/10.1056/ NEJMoa2311330.*

Mackay A. A paradigm for post-COVID-19 fatigue syndrome analogous to ME/CFS. *Front Neurol.* 2021;**12**:701419. *https://doi.org/10.3389/fneur.2021.701419.*

Meinhardt J, Streit S, Dittmayer C, Manitius RV, Radbruch H, Heppner FL. The neurobiology of SARS-CoV-2 infection. *Nat Rev Neurosci.* 2024;**25**(1):30–42. *https://doi. org/10.1038/s41583-023-00769-8.*

Rua C, Raman B, Rodgers CT, Newcombe VFJ, et al. Quantitative susceptibility mapping at 7T in COVID-19: brainstem effects and outcome associations. *Brain.* 2024;**147**(12):4121–30. *https://doi.org/10.1093/brain/awae215.*

Shan ZY, Barnden LR, Kwiatek RA, et al. Neuroimaging characteristics of myalgic encephalomyelitis/chronic fatigue syndrome (ME/CFS): a systematic review. *J Transl Med.* 2020;**18**:335. *https://doi.org/10.1186/s12967-020-02506-6*

Tate WP, Walker MOM, Peppercorn K, Blair ALH, Edgar CD. Towards a better understanding of the complexities of myalgic encephalomyelitis/chronic fatigue syndrome and Long Covid. *Int J Mol Sci.* 2023;**24**(6):5124. *https://doi.org/10.3390/ijms2 4065124.*

Tate W, Walker M, Sweetman E, et al. Molecular mechanisms of neuroinflammation in ME/CFS and Long Covid to sustain disease and promote relapses. *Front Neurol.* 2022;**13**:877772. *https://doi.org/10.3389/fneur.2022.877772.*

Theoharides TC, Cholevas C, Polyzoidis K, Politis A. Long Covid syndrome-associated brain fog and chemofog: luteolin to the rescue. *Biofactors.* 2021;**47**(2):232–41. *https:// doi.org/10.1002/biof.1726.*

5.5 Autonomic nervous system abnormalities

There is robust evidence for autonomic dysfunction in both ME/CFS and Long Covid. This is manifest with symptoms of postural tachycardia (postural orthostatic tachycardia syndrome, POTS) and postural hypotension. Children and young adults are more likely to get vasovagal symptoms. The sensation of air hunger experienced by ME/CFS patients is probably also a result of autonomic dysfunction, although this is not proven. In Long Covid, how much of persisting respiratory symptoms are due to direct lung damage and how much to autonomic dysfunction as in ME/CFS is unknown. However, recent studies from Imperial College London (presented at the European Respiratory Society in 2024) have shown persistent perfusion abnormalities up to 12 months after COVID-19 infection in those who are still symptomatic, even though CT scans are normal. Exercise intolerance was accompanied by evidence of myopericarditis in 46.3% and dysautonomia in only 12%. There were no signs of pulmonary hypertension. ACE levels and anti-phospholipid antibodies were elevated, suggesting the possibility of an ongoing microangiopathy. Lung function was normal apart from a reduced diffusion capacity, which improved slowly over time but did not return to normal. It will be essential to revisit these studies in patients diagnosed with ME/CFS in whom breathlessness is identified to ascertain whether similar mechanisms are at work.

How much of the autonomic problem is due to primary neurological damage and how much to secondary deconditioning is unclear at present. As discussed in section 5.4, there is now MRI evidence for neuroinflammation in the brainstem, which would affect autonomic function, especially breathing. The detection of β2-adrenoreceptor and M3 acetylcholine receptor antibodies may be significant in this regard, as both neurotransmitters are involved in the autonomic nervous system. The presence of these autoantibodies has been used to justify the use of immunoadsorption therapies (see Chapter 9.8). It is noteworthy that autonomic dysfunction is not unique to ME/CFS but is also seen in other conditions associated with marked chronic fatigue, such as primary biliary cirrhosis, hypermobile Ehlers–Danlos syndrome, fibromyalgia, functional bowel and bladder disorders, migraine, and a wide range of other autoimmune and neurological conditions.

Autonomic symptoms are more likely in patients who spend the majority of their time in the horizontal position, as this leads to atrophy of the reflexes normally involved in the control of the cardiovascular seems (pulse and blood pressure) under gravity. This is the same effect as seen in astronauts who spend long periods in zero gravity.

Studies have shown that the cognitive dysfunction in ME/CFS is associated with POTS and not with depression, further evidence that ME/CFS is not 'just' depression.

POTS can usually be diagnosed on a simple active stand test, with both pulse and blood pressure monitored. Tilt table testing will give a more accurate assessment and will allow measurement of the cardiac beat-to-beat variation. Other tests may be used to supplement the basic tests (cold pressor and hand-grip tests). POTS is amenable to treatment, but if drug therapy is required, then this should only be instigated by a physician experienced in the management of POTS (see Chapter 9.14).

POTS itself, even in the absence of other ME/CFS symptoms, is associated with brain fog (cognitive dysfunction) and disturbed sleep, symptoms of irritable bowel, and irritable bladder. Thus, there is considerable overlap between POTS and ME/CFS, as well as other related symptom complexes.

Other cardiac abnormalities have also been documented, such as reduced stroke volume and resting cardiac output, and altered heart rate variability, which are likely to be related to autonomic dysfunction, lowered blood pressure, and inflammation. This can progress to actual heart failure with abnormalities of left ventricular function. Cerebral blood flow is impaired. Patients with Long Covid also have an increased risk of developing cardiovascular disease, including heart failure, myocarditis, pericarditis, endothelial dysfunction, vascular inflammation, and microclots.

Autonomic dysfunction has also been linked to mast cell dysfunction and a skewing of the immune response to a Th2 response in ME/CFS and Long Covid (see section 5.8).

FURTHER READING

Chadda KR, Blakey EE, Huang CL, Jeevaratnam K. Long COVID-19 and postural orthostatic tachycardia syndrome—is dysautonomia to be blamed? *Front Cardiovasc Med.* 2022;**9**:860198. *https://doi.org/10.3389/fcvm.2022.860198.*

Hoad A, Spickett G, Elliott J, Newton J, Postural orthostatic tachycardia syndrome is an under-recognized condition in chronic fatigue syndrome, *QJM.* 2008;**101**(12):961–5. *https://doi.org/10.1093/qjmed/hcn123.*

Natelson B, Brunjes D, Mancini D. Chronic fatigue syndrome and cardiovascular disease: JACC state-of-the-art review. *J Am Coll Cardiol.* 2021;**78**(10):1056–67. *https://doi.org/ 10.1016/j.jacc.2021.06.045.*

Newton JL, Okonkwo O, Sutcliffe K, Seth A, Shin J, Jones DE. Symptoms of autonomic dysfunction in chronic fatigue syndrome. *QJM.* 2007;**100**(8):519–26. *https://doi.org/ 10.1093/qjmed/hcm057.*

Nelson MJ, Bahl JS, Buckley JD, Thomson RL, Davison K. Evidence of altered cardiac autonomic regulation in myalgic encephalomyelitis/chronic fatigue syndrome: a systematic review and meta-analysis. *Medicine (Baltimore).* 2019;**98**(43):e17600. *https:// doi.org/10.1097/MD.0000000000017600.*

Robinson LJ, Gallagher P, Watson S, Pearce R, Finkelmeyer A, Maclachlan L, Newton JL. Impairments in cognitive performance in chronic fatigue syndrome are common, not related to co-morbid depression but do associate with autonomic dysfunction. *PLoS One.* 2019;**14**(2):e0210394. *https://doi.org/10.1371/journal.pone.0210394.*

Słomko J, Estévez-López F, Kujawski S, et al. Autonomic phenotypes in chronic fatigue syndrome (CFS) are associated with illness severity: a cluster analysis. *J Clin Med.* 2020;**9**(8):2531. *https://doi.org/10.3390/jcm9082531.*

5.6 Endocrine abnormalities

Endocrine abnormalities have been described in ME/CFS. These include abnormalities of T3 and rT3, low testosterone and oestrogen, and sometimes low cortisol. Whether these abnormalities are primary or secondary is unclear. Most studies have not shown significant benefits from hormone replacement, although there has been advocacy over the years for treatments with thyroid hormones, sex hormones, and steroids. This may include the use of triiodothyronine (T3) or thyroid extracts (Armour), which are unstandardized. In the UK, a prescription from a General Medical Council (GMC) registered doctor is required for thyroid extracts. Excessive or inappropriate use of thyroid hormones or thyroid extracts can make symptoms worse and contribute to a persistent raised pulse rate. It is important to ascertain whether a patient is taking any thyroid extracts or other prescribed thyroid replacements if there is an inappropriately raised pulse, before embarking on other investigations.

More recently it has been suggested that the neuroinflammatory process that has been described in both ME/CFS and Long Covid has a direct impact on the HPA, leading to dysregulation of hormone production. It has also been suggested that there may be an autoimmune element to the hypothalamic dysfunction. These include antibodies to β2-adrenoreceptors and M3/M4 cholinergic receptors, both of which are expressed in the hypothalamus. PET scanning of patients with ME/CFS and antibodies to cholinergic receptors has shown a reduction of the ligand in the hypothalamus. The normal increase in morning cortisol is absent in patients with Long Covid. If this was significant, then it would be expected that hormone replacement might have a positive impact on at least some of the symptoms, but this does not seem to be the case, at least with the available evidence so far. Similar evidence of low cortisol and lack of response to steroid replacement has been seen in ME/CFS.

Unless there are clinical features suggestive of hormonal deficiency, then routine endocrine screening apart from thyroid function is not indicated. Patients with marked hypotension, especially postural, should have morning cortisol checked. Any suspicious features, either clinically or on initial investigation, should lead to an endocrine opinion on further investigation such as a short Synacthen test.

To confuse matters further, it is possible that some endocrine abnormalities have been present, but undetected, prior to the development of ME/CFS or Long Covid and are only identified once investigation is undertaken. These may be contributory to symptoms or may simply be incidental findings. They may also be risk factors for the development of the diseases.

FURTHER READING

Bansal R, Gubbi S, Koch CA. COVID-19 and chronic fatigue syndrome: an endocrine perspective. *J Clin Transl Endocrinol.* 2022;**27**:100284. *https://doi.org/10.1016/j.jcte.2021.100284.*

De Bellis A, Bellastella G, Pernice V, et al. Hypothalamic-pituitary autoimmunity and related impairment of hormone secretions in chronic fatigue syndrome. *J Clin Endocrinol Metab.* 2021;106(12):e5147–55. *https://doi.org/10.1210/clinem/dgab429.*

Nakano Y, Sunada N, Tokumasu K, et al. Occult endocrine disorders newly diagnosed in patients with post-COVID-19 symptoms. *Sci Rep* 2024;14:5446. *https://doi.org/10.1038/s41598-024-55526-3.*

5.7 Mitochondrial abnormalities

There is quite a long history of association of ME/CFS with mitochondrial dysfunction and more recently in Long Covid. What is not clear is whether the abnormalities are primary or secondary. Careful studies of muscle metabolism in ME/CFS have demonstrated abnormal muscle metabolism, with excessive acidosis and abnormal mitochondrial function.

A meta-analysis of the research evidence for mitochondrial abnormalities in ME/CFS concluded that inconsistencies across the studies made it difficult to conclude beyond reasonable doubt that there was an underlying mitochondrial defect in ME/CFS and the evidence did not differentiate between a primary pathogenic cause and secondary changes. It has been suggested recently that the abnormalities of mitochondria, through the release of their DNA, in the brain may contribute to neuroinflammation through stimulation of microglial production of IL-1β. Studies of mitochondria in the periphery may therefore not accurately reflect the involvement of mitochondria at selective sites. Studies have not indicated any fundamental abnormalities in the genetic make-up of mitochondria in ME/CFS patients.

An increase in the expression of the mammalian target of rapamycin complex 1 (mTORC1) has been identified in ME/CFS. This protein is involved in regulating the translation of mitochondrial proteins. Poor synthesis of adenosine triphosphate (ATP) has been noted in mitochondria in patients with ME/CFS. Elevated levels of WASF3 (a member of the Wiskott–Aldrich syndrome protein family) have been identified in ME/CFS muscle cells. This protein interferes with the mitochondrial protein assembly required for the synthesis of ATP. Overproduction of this protein in the muscles of transgenic mice caused increased fatigue on exertion.

Co-enzyme Q10 is thought to be crucial for mitochondrial function, and there is some limited evidence to suggest deficiency of CoQ10 in ME/CFS. This has led to several trials of this compound, often with nicotinamide adenine dinucleotide (NADH) (also an important molecule in mitochondria), as a treatment for ME/CFS, with apparent benefit to fatigue, cognitive function, quality of life and sleep. As neither of these compounds appears to have any major side effects, then a trial of treatment may be beneficial. However, the benefit does not automatically indicate that the mitochondria are at fault as the compounds may have other effects.

Oxidative stress has also been proposed as part of the pathogenesis of ME/CFS and Long Covid. Redox abnormalities have been described in both conditions, and levels of antioxidants are reported to be reduced and pro-oxidants are increased. These changes involve complex changes in small molecules and impaired energy metabolism in mitochondria (Paul et al., 2021). The same abnormalities in the redox state in ME/CFS and Long Covid confirm that these conditions are likely to have the same underlying pathology and do suggest some possible avenues for treatments. Anecdotal evidence suggests benefit from supplementation, but robust clinical trials have not yet been conducted. Because there are multiple potential antioxidants, trials of oral single compounds or even combinations have been less than dramatic. Finding the right combination and working out the best time for administration will take longer. In some similar scenarios with fatigue and muscle damage (associated with intense exercise) with low levels of antioxidants, supplementation has not been proven to be beneficial and may even be harmful.

FURTHER READING

Booth NE, Myhill S, McLaren-Howard J. Mitochondrial dysfunction and the pathophysiology of myalgic encephalomyelitis/chronic fatigue syndrome (ME/CFS). *Int J Clin Exp Med*. 2012;5(3):208.

Castro-Marrero J, Segundo MJ, Lacasa M, Martinez-Martinez A, Sentañes RS, Alegre-Martin J. Effect of dietary coenzyme Q10 plus NADH supplementation on fatigue perception and health-related quality of life in individuals with myalgic encephalomyelitis/chronic fatigue syndrome: a prospective, randomized, double-blind, placebo-controlled trial. *Nutrients*. 2021;13(8):2658. *https://doi.org/10.3390/nu13082658*.

Holden S, Maksoud R, Eaton-Fitch N, Cabanas H, Staines D, Marshall-Gradisnik S. A systematic review of mitochondrial abnormalities in myalgic encephalomyelitis/chronic fatigue syndrome/systemic exertion intolerance disease. *J Transl Med*. 2020;18(1):290. *https://doi.org/10.1186/s12967-020-02452-3*.

Maes M, Mihaylova I, Kubera M, Uytterhoeven M, Vrydags N, Bosmans E. Coenzyme Q10 deficiency in myalgic encephalomyelitis/chronic fatigue syndrome (ME/CFS) is related to fatigue, autonomic and neurocognitive symptoms and is another risk factor explaining the early mortality in ME/CFS due to cardiovascular disorder. *Neuro Endocrinol Lett*. 2009;30(4):470–6.

Paul BD, Lemle MD, Komaroff AL, Snyder SH. Redox imbalance links COVID-19 and myalgic encephalomyelitis/chronic fatigue syndrome. *Proc Natl Acad Sci*. 2021;118(34):e2024358118. *https://doi.org/10.1073/pnas.2024358118*.

Tomas C, Elson JL, Strassheim V, Newton JL, Walker M. The effect of myalgic encephalomyelitis/chronic fatigue syndrome (ME/CFS) severity on cellular bioenergetic function. *PLoS One*. 2020;15(4):e0231136. *https://doi.org/10.1371/journal.pone.0231136*.

5.8 Immunological abnormalities

The genetic studies discussed earlier suggest that there may be an immunogenetic background predisposing to the development of ME/CFS and Long Covid, although this is quite clearly polygenic. The abnormalities may predispose to an abnormal response to the initiating infection and/or lead to an inappropriate cytokine response or an inappropriately long cytokine response that is not switched off by the normal immunological control mechanisms. It seems likely that the primary site of this inappropriate response is in the brain, probably related to microglial activation. The persistence of SARS-CoV2 in the brain may be a driver to this in Long Covid. Thus, it seems likely that the immune system is contributing to a chronic neuroinflammatory process

The concept of brain inflammation has a long history, going back to the Royal Free Hospital outbreak, which led to the original name of myalgic encephalomyelitis. Investigations at the time, bearing in mind the scientific techniques available, were consistent with neuroinflammation following symptoms highly suggestive of an infection. This was buried by the McEvedy & Beard paper in the *BMJ* in 1970, which described the episode as one of epidemic hysteria. This sadly led to the widespread belief that ME/CFS was a psychiatric, not a medical, illness. Reevaluation of the episode, including re-interview of survivors, concluded that the illness was most in keeping with an acute infectious illness that was not just confined to the hospital but affected the local populations as well and many survivors had long-term illness consistent with ME/CFS.

Autoantibodies against the β2-adrenergic receptor and the acetylcholine M3 and M4 receptors have been described in ME/CFS. These receptors are deemed to be important in mediating vasodilation, so it is hypothesized that the antibodies may block vasodilation in response to exercise and, therefore, create relative hypoxemia in muscle. It has also been suggested that these autoantibodies may contribute to the cardiac abnormalities identified in ME/CFS, including rate problems and cardiac muscle dysfunction. This would correlate with the finding of abnormal cellular energetics in exercising muscles from patients with ME/CFS findings that would be consistent with relative hypoxemia. The β2-adrenergic receptors also mediate airway vasodilation, so blocking antibodies might lead to the narrowing of the airway and perhaps contribute to the 'air hunger' described by patients. It has suggested that removal of the autoantibodies by apheresis leads to benefit. There does not appear to be any intrathecal synthesis of these autoantibodies, leaving an open question about whether they have a role in neurological inflammation. Peripherally synthesized antibodies will only enter the nervous system if there is a breakdown of the blood–brain barrier, such as may occur in any inflammatory process affecting the brain. However, it is hypothesized that these antibodies may contribute to disordered hypothalamic function (see earlier).

In the context of COVID-19 infection, antiphospholipid antibodies have been described and seem to be associated with more severe disease and with the presence of intracerebral clotting. Whether there is a direct or indirect linkage to Long Covid is not yet known. Antiphospholipid autoantibodies have been tentatively linked to POTS, but not specifically to ME/CFS. The primary anti-phospholipid syndrome is most typically associated with recurrent peripheral and central nervous system (CNS) thromboses, and like any chronic illness, fatigue may be an element. Infection may be a trigger for these antibodies. So far, there is nothing to suggest that anti-phospholipid antibodies play a direct role in the ongoing pathogenesis of ME/CFS, although if they were transiently triggered at the onset of the illness by an infection, causing cerebral dysfunction, but then disappearing, this would not be picked up due to the delay in assessing patients with ME/CFS.

Anti-nuclear antibodies have been described in both ME/CFS and Long Covid, but these do not appear to be a consistent feature. Infections of all types may be associated with the transient appearance of anti-nuclear antibodies. Adenovirus infection is particularly associated with the appearance of anti-nuclear antibodies. The interest in mitochondrial dysfunction begs the question as to whether anti-mitochondrial antibodies might be involved, but there does not appear to be any evidence for this in ME/CFS. Primary biliary cirrhosis, which is associated with anti-mitochondrial antibodies, is strongly associated with chronic fatigue and autonomic problems (POTS, vasovagal syncope), while chronic active hepatitis, another liver disease which is associated with anti-smooth muscle antibodies, does not appear to have fatigue or autonomic dysfunction as a significant part of the symptomatology.

Studies of immune cells in ME/CFS and Long Covid have shown that their patterns of gene transcription are highly abnormal, with unregulated production of some immune mediators (IL-8 and TNFα) and down-regulation of others. Multiple genes have been identified, including FOXN1, PRDX3, SUCLA2, TYK2, among others, but patterns of activation/repression are complex and difficult to map to symptoms and progression. It is likely that patterns of immune gene expression will vary depending on the stage of the illness and the predominant symptoms, and possibly to the nature of the triggering organism.

Abnormalities of humoral and cellular immune function have been described. It is unclear whether these are simply secondary to the illness or play a role in the genesis of the illness. Abnormalities of serum immunoglobulins (IgG subclasses) have been reported and B lymphocytes subsets may be altered. There is no convincing evidence, however, to link ME/CFS and Long Covid to a specific immune deficiency. Unusually severe responses to common organisms have been linked with specific gene defects, for example, in HSV encephalitis, so it is possible that there is a very specific immunological deficiency that predisposes to ME/CFS. The genetic studies have not so far identified any such single gene link. Proteomic studies have shown evidence of antigen-driven clonal B cell expansion, which may be linked to autoantibody production, discussed earlier. T and B cell subsets and NK cell numbers and function are altered. NK cell cytotoxicity is reduced by poor function in the TRPM3 ion channel, which is essential to NK cytotoxicity. Naltrexone, which is sometimes recommended in low doses for the treatment of ME/CFS, appears to improve NK cell function by acting on this molecule. Whether or how this is relevant to the pathology or treatment of ME/CFS or Long Covid is uncertain. There is an increase in activated (CD38+) CD8+ cytotoxic cells. CD8+ T cells show a severe deficiency in the capacity to produce IFN-γ and TNFα in both ME/CFS and Long Covid. It has been suggested that over time, the T-cell profiles show evidence of T-cell exhaustion. There is evidence that both an increase and a decrease in regulatory T cells, which may be explained by the stage at which patients were studied and the nature of the triggering event. B lymphocytes from patients with ME/CFS have shown reduced numbers of mitochondria, delayed loss of CD24, and an increased expression of CD38. Whether this is cause or effect is unknown, but it is evidence of persistent immune dysregulation. Monocyte function is disturbed with abnormal differentiation and migration.

Evidence for persistent low-grade systemic inflammation in Long Covid has been postulated and attributed to elevated proportions of CD14+ CD16+ and CD14lowCD16+ monocytes producing TNF-α, IL-1β, and Il-6. Similar changes are seen in acute COVID-19 and normally disappear, but persist in patients going to develop Long Covid.

Platelet function is also altered. These changes appear worse after symptom provocation by exercise, confirming that the described post-exertional malaise is accompanied by significant immunological changes.

A recent paper in *Science* has shown increased activation of the complement system of a persistent nature in patients with Long Covid. This included elevated levels of soluble C5bC6 and of the terminal complement complex (TCC C5–C9). Low levels of anti-thrombin 3 were accompanied by increased levels of cleavage by thrombin, which in turn elevated the TCC. Platelet activation levels were increased. There was also antibody activation of TCC, linked to increased levels of antibodies to cytomegalovirus (CMV) and EBV (part of an anamnestic response). Overall, this suggests that in Long Covid there is a continuing process of thromboinflammation and complement-mediated tissue damage. As noted earlier, the role of complement in microglial function may link the complement abnormalities to neuroinflammation. Similar studies need to be carried out in early stage ME/CFS, and the duration of these abnormalities needs to be clarified. If it is shown to be a long-term phenomenon, then testing would potentially be a useful marker of disease activity.

Cytokine patterns in ME/CFS are variable. Increased production of pro-inflammatory cytokines (IL-1A, IL-17α, TNF-α) and anti-inflammatory cytokines (IL-1RA, IL-4, IL-13) are seen in the early phases of the illness up to 3 years. Early attempts at using therapeutic doses of single cytokines in ME/CFS in the 1990s led to deterioration in symptoms and were abandoned. A recent study on a single patient with severe ME/CFS (bed-bound) and hypermobility spectrum disorder found significant skewing of cytokine responses to Th2 and suggested that this might link with mast cell activation, POTS, and small fibre neuropathy.

Overall, the evidence suggests that disordered homeostasis of the immune system occurs early in ME/CFS and Long Covid and leads to the production of autoantibodies, abnormal T, B NK cell, and microglial function, disordered cytokine production with excess inflammatory cytokines and complement activation. These changes appear to directly affect areas of the brain, interfering with cognition, and endocrine function. The most recent studies confirm that the immunological changes are very similar in both ME/CFS and Long Covid.

FURTHER READING

Altmann DM, Whettlock EM, Liu S, Arachchillage DJ, Boyton RJ. The immunology of Long Covid. *Nat Rev Immunol.* 2023;23(10):618–34. *https://doi.org/10.1038/s41 577-023-00904-7.*

Bansal AS, Kraneveld AD, Oltra E, Carding S. What causes ME/CFS: the role of the dysfunctional immune system and viral infections. *J Immuno Allerg.* 2022;3(2):1–15. *https://doi.org/10.37191/Mapsci-2582-6549-3(2)-033.*

Cervia-Hasler C, Brüningk SC, Hoch T, et al. Persistent complement dysregulation with signs of thromboinflammation in active Long Covid. *Science.* 2024;383;eadg7942. *https://doi.org/10.1126/science.adg7942.*

Gravelsina S, Vilmane A, Svirskis S, et al. Biomarkers in the diagnostic algorithm of myalgic encephalomyelitis/chronic fatigue syndrome. *Front Immunol.* 2022;13:928945. *https:// doi.org/10.3389/fimmu.2022.928945.*

Jahanbani F, Sing JC, Maynard RD, et al. Longitudinal cytokine and multi-modal health data of an extremely severe ME/CFS patient with HSD reveals insights into immunopathology, and disease severity. *Front Immunol.* 2024;15:1369295. *https://doi. org/10.3389/fimmu.2024.1369295.*

Peppercorn K, Edgar CD, Kleffmann T, et al. A pilot study on the immune cell proteome of Long Covid patients shows changes to physiological pathways similar to those in myalgic encephalomyelitis/chronic fatigue syndrome. *Sci Rep.* 2023;13:22068. *https://doi.org/ 10.1038/s41598-023-49402-9.*

Theoharides TC, Twahir A, Kempuraj D. Mast cells in the autonomic nervous system and potential role in disorders with dysautonomia and neuroinflammation. *Ann Allergy Asthma Immunol.* 2024;132(4):440–54. *https://doi.org/10.1016/j.anai.2023.10.032.*

Vu LT, Ahmed F, Zhu H, et al. Single-cell transcriptomics of the immune system in ME/ CFS at baseline and following symptom provocation. *Cell Rep Med.* 2024;5(1):101373. *https://doi.org/10.1016/j.xcrm.2023.101373.*

Wirth K, Scheibenbogen C. A unifying hypothesis of the pathophysiology of myalgic encephalomyelitis/chronic fatigue syndrome (ME/CFS): recognitions from the finding of autoantibodies against ß2-adrenergic receptors. *Autoimmun Rev.* 2020;19(6):102527. *https://doi.org/10.1016/j.autrev.2020.102527.*

5.9 Clotting abnormalities

Acute SARS-CoV2 and Long Covid have both been associated with clotting disorders, and it is considered that cerebral microthrombi might contribute to some of the neurological damage and possibly other organ damage. Up until recently, there had been no studies on ME/CFS. New studies have, however, confirmed abnormalities are present in ME/CFS patients too. Fibrinaloid clots and a generalized hypercoagulability in association with an inflammatory state are key features in Long Covid. There has been debate about the nature of the 'micro clots': they do not appear to involve platelets, just fibrin and fibrinogen, together with amyloid protein. However, hyperactivated platelets can also be seen in Long Covid. For ME/CFS and Long Covid, it is unclear whether these are persistent features long term, or whether they are just part of the initiation phase of the illness. The precise role of these 'microclots' in the pathogenesis is equally uncertain. Plasmapheresis to remove the 'micro clots' has been used, although the evidence to support this is weak (Fox et al., 1996). Another unanswered question is whether clinical relapse is associated with a resurgence of clotting abnormalities. Further research is required to ascertain exactly what role clotting abnormalities play in the genesis and persistence of fatigue in ME/CFS and Long Covid.

Autoantibodies to endothelial cells have also been detected in Long Covid patients, but the significance of these is uncertain.

FURTHER READING

Fox T, Hunt BJ, Ariens RA, et al. Plasmapheresis to remove amyloid fibrin (ogen) particles for treating the post-COVID-19 condition. *Cochrane Database Syst Rev.* 1996;2023(7). *https://doi.org//10.1002/14651858.CD015775.*

Nunes JM, Kruger A, Proal A, Kell DB, Pretorius E. The occurrence of hyperactivated platelets and fibrinaloid microclots in myalgic encephalomyelitis/chronic fatigue syndrome (ME/CFS). *Pharmaceuticals (Basel).* 2022;15(8):931. *https://doi.org/10.3390/ph15080931.*

Pretorius E, Venter C, Laubscher GJ, et al. Prevalence of symptoms, comorbidities, fibrin amyloid microclots and platelet pathology in individuals with Long Covid/post-acute sequelae of COVID-19 (PASC). *Cardiovasc Diabetol.* 2022;21(1):148. *https://doi.org/10.1186/s12933-022-01579-5.*

5.10 Gut microbiome and associated disorders

There is now increasing data available on abnormalities of the gut microbiome in ME/CFS, which shows that patients have a reduced diversity of gut microbiome, compared to healthy individuals. Butyrate-producing bacteria (*Faecalibacterium prausnitzii (F. prausnitzii)* and *Eubacterium rectale*) appear to be reduced; the lower the levels of these bacteria, the worse the symptoms of ME/CFS (NIH, 2023). Butyrate is a bacterial metabolite that is associated with gut health and actually provides 70% of the energy requirements for the gut mucosal cells and mucosal immune cells. Increases in other bacteria that have been associated with auto-immune disease and inflammatory bowel disease have also been recorded. It has been suggested that the alterations may be sufficiently robust as to constitute a biological signature for ME/CFS and aid diagnosis.

Reduction in bacteria involved in tryptophan metabolism (kynurenine pathway) has also been noted. This pathway has a significant role in linking the bowel to inflammation in the brain. Disturbance of tryptophan metabolism has a profound effect on immune function and contributes to fatigue. This pathway is also involved in the synthesis of nicotinamide adenine dinucleotide (NAD), an essential molecule involved in cellular energy supply, supplementation of which, in combination with co-enzyme Q10, has been shown to improve ME/CFS symptoms (see section 5.7).

The concept of a 'leaky gut' contributing to ME/CFS has been around for a long while. Studies of the microbiome suggest that reduced butyrate production may indeed lead to gut leakiness. This leads onto the possibility that the leakiness enables excessive amounts of bacterial lipopolysaccharide to reach the deeper layers and stimulate an inflammatory reaction. Whether this scenario is a major contributor to fatigue remains as yet unproven. Changes in the gut microflora and increased leakiness may increase D-lactic acid levels: this is thought to cause neurological symptoms. However, the use of probiotics made no difference to the production of D-lactate.

Abnormalities of the gut microbiome have also been described in patients with COVID-19 infection and Long Covid. As in ME/CFS, the pathological significance of these changes is not known. Equally unknown is whether attempts to manipulate the microbiome are beneficial. It is unlikely that standard probiotic over-the-counter supplements contain the correct bacteria to resolve the problem.

A doctoral thesis has studied the IgG response to gut bacteria in ME/CFS and found that patients had impaired IgG responses to gut bacteria, compared to household controls. This is suggestive that changes in flora may be directly influencing immunological reactivity (Seton et al., 2023).

Overall, at present it is unclear whether changes in the microbiome play a primary pathological role, are secondary to the illness but have a role in perpetuating the illness or are epiphenomena that do not impact the illness. Of these, the evidence is more in favour of the first or second, and the changes seem unlikely to be insignificant epiphenomena.

A further complication has been added to hypotheses about the impact of the gut microbiome, and that is the role of the gut virome. Just as the gut is teeming with bacteria, it is also teeming with viruses, 97% of which are phages, that is, viruses that infect bacteria. These bacteriophages appear to play a key role in the regulation of the microbiome, as well as being one mechanism for transferring genes (e.g. antibiotic resistance) between bacteria. Every individual's virome is unique. Research is underway to assess the impact of these viruses on brain function and already there is suggestive evidence that bacteriophages of the Caudovirales family have an impact on cognitive function and on stress responses (Ritz et al., 2024). The impact of this on ME/CFS and Long Covid remains to be assessed.

ME/CFS patients all have symptoms of irritable bowel syndrome, and food intolerance is common. Typically, wheat is associated with symptoms but sometimes all members of the FODMAPS group of foods are associated with increased symptoms. As irritable bowel syndrome (IBS) is also thought to be linked to alteration of the gut microflora, this would link with these findings. It is established that the gut microbiome changes in response to diet, so a trial of wheat avoidance or more complex dietary changes under dietician guidance is not unreasonable. However, there is an enormous amount of alternative information available on the internet about food intolerances and ME/CFS, and many sites offering food intolerance testing. Much of this testing is not based on robust science, especially variants of Vega testing. It is important to ensure that patients understand the limitations of this type of testing and are discouraged from spending large quantities of money on tests of unproven value. Equally, there are risks from the implementation of severely restrictive diets. There is no indication that the *primary* cause of ME/CFS is food intolerance or allergy.

Long Covid is also associated with an increased prevalence of irritable bowel symptoms., but not functional dyspepsia. Gastrointestinal symptoms during the acute episode of COVID-19 increase the risk of developing irritable bowel disease subsequently. There caveats about treatment for IBS in ME/CFS apply equally to Long Covid.

It has been suggested that there is a functional deficiency of vitamin B_{12} in ME/CFS. Why this should occur is not yet understood. Small studies have shown that symptoms may improve on supplements even if the serum B12 levels are normal in some but not all patients.

FURTHER READING

Guo C, Che X, Briese T, et al. Deficient butyrate-producing capacity in the gut microbiome is associated with bacterial network disturbances and fatigue symptoms in ME/CFS. *Cell Host Microbe.* 2023;**31**:288–304. *https://doi.org/10.1016/j.chom.2023.01.004.*

Hilpert K, Mikut R. Is there a connection between gut microbiome dysbiosis occurring in COVID-19 patients and post-COVID-19 symptoms? *Front Microbiol.* 2021;**12**:732838. *https://doi.org/10.3389/fmicb.2021.732838.*

König RS, Albrich WC, Kahlert CR, et al. The gut microbiome in myalgic encephalomyelitis (ME)/chronic fatigue syndrome (CFS). *Front Immunol.* 2022;**12**:628741. *https://doi.org/10.3389/fimmu.2021.628741.*

Lupo GF, Rocchetti G, Lucini L, et al. Potential role of microbiome in chronic fatigue syndrome/myalgic encephalomyelits (ME/CFS). *Sci Rep.* 2021;**11**(1):7043. *https://doi.org/10.1038/s41598-021-86425-6.*

Maes M, Leunis JC. Normalization of leaky gut in chronic fatigue syndrome (CFS) is accompanied by a clinical improvement: effects of age, duration of illness and the translocation of LPS from Gram-negative bacteria. Neuro Endocrinol Lett. 2008 Dec;**29**(6):902–10. PMID: 19112401.

Marasco G, Cremon C, Barbaro MR, et al. Post COVID-19 irritable bowel syndrome. *Gut.* 2023;**72**(3):484–92. *https://doi.org/10.1136/gutjnl-2022-328483.*

National Institute of Health (NIH). Studies find that microbiome changes may be a signature for ME/CFS. *News Releases 2023. https://www.nih.gov/news-events/news-releases/studies-find-microbiome-changes-may-be-signature-mecfs.*

Regland B, Forsmark S, Halaouate L, et al. Response to vitamin B_{12} and folic acid in myalgic encephalomyelitis and fibromyalgia. *PLoS One.* 2015;**10**(4):e0124648. *https://doi.org/10.1371/journal.pone.0124648.*

Ritz NL, Draper LA, Bastiaanssen TF, et al. The gut virome is associated with stress-induced changes in behaviour and immune responses in mice. *Nat Microbiol.* 2024;9(2):359–76. *https://doi.org/10.1038/s41564-023-01564-y.*

Seton KA, Defernez M, Telatin A, et al. Investigating antibody reactivity to the intestinal microbiome in severe myalgic encephalomyelitis/chronic fatigue syndrome (ME/CFS): a feasibility study. *Int J Mol Sci.* 2023;24(20):15316. *https://doi.org/10.3390/ijms242015 316.*

Stallmach A, Quickert S, Puta C, Reuken PA. The gastrointestinal microbiota in the development of ME/CFS: a critical view and potential perspectives. *Front Immunol.* 2024;15:1352744. *https://doi.org/10.3389/fimmu.2024.1352744.*

Wang JH, Choi Y, Lee JS, Hwang SJ, Gu J, Son CG. Clinical evidence of the link between gut microbiome and myalgic encephalomyelitis/chronic fatigue syndrome: a retrospective review. *Eur J Med Res.* 2024;29(1):148. *https://doi.org/10.1186/s40 001-024-01747-1.*

5.11 **Psychiatric**

As discussed in the introduction to this chapter, it is quite clear that psychological issues predispose to the development of ME/CFS. There are studies confirming that there is an excess of major life events/stressors, preceding the development of ME/CFS. These can be other serious illnesses (either personal or family/friends), unemployment, separation or divorce, and bereavement. In the diagnostic assessment, one needs to be quite clear that these events are not sufficiently severe to have triggered a post-traumatic stress disorder, as this too can be associated with severe fatigue, but needs a different approach to therapy. Military or ex-military personnel who have served in conflict zones are particularly likely to develop post-traumatic stress disorder (PTSD), but civilians who have experienced traumatic events are just as likely to develop it. There is a specific scoring system for this.[2]

In this context, therefore, the extreme stress that NHS staff experienced working through the COVID-19 pandemic is very likely to be a contributory factor in their susceptibility to develop Long Covid when infected with the virus. Healthcare workers during and after the pandemic have clearly suffered burnout, which can mimic ME/CFS or Long Covid (see Chapter 4.2).

Notwithstanding this, there is still a strongly held view among psychiatrists and psychologists that ME/CFS represent any or all of the following: a variant of anxiety and/or depression, somatization, or simply factitious illness. Medical perceptions of the illness were disproportionately affected by the McEvedy & Beard paper referred to previously. This lack of belief still stretches into other medical disciplines and into general practice. Hopefully, the impact of 'Long Covid' may educate some unbelievers that ME/CFS, too, is a very real medical illness.

---

[2] For more information, see US Department of Veterans Affairs, 'PTSD Checklist for *DSM-5* (PCL-5)', *https://www.ptsd.va.gov/professional/assessment/adult-sr/ptsd-checklist.asp*

The pernicious tendency of the medical profession to assume that any patient with 'medically unexplained symptoms' is either mad or bad or both has a profoundly negative effect not only on the patient but also on the prospects for research. A historical example of this concerns gastric ulcers. At the beginning of the twentieth century, all the way through until the 1990s, it was the belief that gastric ulcers were related to the patient's inadequate personality. The discovery at the end of the twentieth century that gastric ulcers were almost all caused by infection of the stomach lining with the bacterium *Helicobacter*, which could easily be treated and cured with a combination of acid-suppressing treatment combined with two antibiotics. No one now would dream of suggesting that patients with gastric ulcers have an abnormal personality which has caused their ulcer! Any abnormal personality traits in patients with gastric ulcers were undoubtedly secondary to the chronic and debilitating pain of an untreated gastric ulcer. I suspect that doctors in 20–50 years' time, when the cause of ME/CFS is fully known and a curative treatment established, will look back in horror at the attribution of a psychological/psychiatric cause for the illness.

The power of the psychiatry/psychology lobby, certainly in the 1990s and early 2000s, meant that ME/CFS was not taken seriously. Many patients were simply told they were depressed. While any patient with long-term chronic illness may become depressed and anxious because of their radically changed circumstances, this does not mean that all of their illness is due to depression and anxiety. Many patients were given anti-depressants, which were not effective in treating the associated fatigue, although they may have been less depressed and anxious about it. The underlying symptoms, however, rarely changed. Evidence has been collected that focusing on the biopsychosocial model of ME/CFS negatively impacts physicians and biases their care away from the identification and management of physical symptoms.

Depression and anxiety or other psychiatric illnesses can be a cause of fatigue and other typical ME/CFS symptoms and form part of the differential diagnosis, which must be considered at the outset. Studies of the brain using MRI imaging, PET scanning, and electroencephalogram (EEG), have shown distinct and reproducible differences between chronic depression and ME/CFS, making it unlikely that ME/CFS is just depression. Cytokines released during the process of neuroinflammation described earlier (in particular IL-6) can have profound effects on both mood and cognition.

Having said all this, it is not surprising that patients with ME/CFS, especially where the social and financial consequences are severe, become depressed and anxious due to their illness. Recognition and treatment of this is important, but this is secondary, not primary, depression. When anti-depressants are used in this context it is important that both patient and doctor recognize that the drugs will not 'cure' the fatigue but will help them cope with the consequences better: happier but still fatigued. This has important implications for the management.

CHAPTER 5

In the context of 'psychiatric' illness it is becoming more apparent that many acute psychiatric problems may actually be caused by autoimmune brain inflammation (encephalitis). There are regular stories of patients with acute and severe behavioural disturbance (psychosis) being sectioned under the Mental Health Act and treated intensively with anti-psychotic drugs, when in fact they have a treatable and reversible autoimmune encephalitis. This actually extends to schizophrenia, a major psychiatric illness, where the latest research shows that some patients at least have an immunological, not psychiatric, problem. If this is generalizable finding, it will have huge implications for psychiatry.

FURTHER READING

Geraghty K. The negative impact of the psychiatric model of chronic fatigue syndrome on doctors' understanding and management of the illness. *Fatigue: Biomed Health Behav.* 2020;8(3):167–80. *https://doi.org/10.1080/21641846.2020.1834295.*

Gangadin SS, Enthoven AD, van Beveren NJ, Laman JD, Sommer IE. Immune dysfunction in schizophrenia spectrum disorders. *Ann Rev Clin Psychol.* 2024;20(1):229–57. *https://doi.org/10.1146/annurev-clinpsy-081122-013201.*

Grain R, Lally J, Stubbs B, et al. Autoantibodies against voltage-gated potassium channel and glutamic acid decarboxylase in psychosis: a systematic review, meta-analysis, and case series. *Psychiatry Clin Neurosci.* 2017;71:678–89. *https://doi.org/10.1111/pcn.12543.*

Sanal-Hayes NE, Mclaughlin M, Hayes LD, Berry EC, Sculthorpe NF. Examining well-being and cognitive function in people with Long Covid and ME/CFS, and age-matched healthy controls: a case-case-control study. *Am J Med.* 2024. *https://doi.org/10.1016/j.amjmed.2024.04.041.*

Watanabe, Y. PET/SPECT/MRI/fMRI studies in the myalgic encephalomyelitis/chronic fatigue syndrome. In: Dierckx RA, Otte A, de Vries EFJ, van Waarde A, Sommer IE, eds. *PET and SPECT in psychiatry.* Springer, 2021: 985–1001. *https://doi.org/10.1007/978-3-030-57231-0_32.*

5.12 Psychosomatic and somatization

The description of an illness as psychosomatic implies that it is all in the mind. Most fatigued patients, because of what they have read, are terrified that when they report their symptoms to healthcare professionals, their illness will be dismissed as 'all in the mind', in the sense of being made up. The undoubted role of inflammation within the brain in ME/CFS means that in a more scientific sense, ME/CFS and Long Covid are a disorder of the brain and perhaps the mind, whatever that is. It is important that healthcare professionals spell out that 'all in the mind' is not the same as 'made up'. As discussed in the introduction to this chapter, it is clear that major psychosocial stress plays an important role in predisposing to the onset of ME/CFS and probably Long Covid, but again this linkage does not indicate that either disease is psychosomatic. Studies comparing

ME/CFS and Long Covid have confirmed the congruence of the psychosocial as well as physical symptom backgrounds.

Somatization is something slightly different, whereby severe psychological stress presents as mainly severe physical symptoms. Then physical symptoms are usually not typical of a true physical disorder, for example, the apparent inability to move a leg, when testing shows that the brain, nerves, and muscles are all working normally. This is not usually a wilful refusal to move the leg but an unconscious block, often without true awareness. There is often a specific gain for the patient through avoidance of painful scenarios, attention-seeking from friends and family, or more subtle gains; for example, bringing warring parents together. While fatigue may be an element, this is usually less of an issue than physical symptoms.

Both psychosomatic illness and somatization are clearly defined and different to the ME/CFS and Long Covid. In my experience, true factitious illness, where the illness is deliberately and completely made up, is unusual in the context of ME/CFS. Here there is inevitably a major gain from illness, usually financial (benefit fraud). Occasionally, patients with true ME/CFS get caught up in benefit or insurance fraud investigations, which adds further to their stress. Where the diagnosis is a clearcut one of ME/CFS, doctors should provide appropriate support to patients that confirm their illness and their functional capacity. Because it is difficult to know from a clinic consultation just how disabled a person is by their illness, I introduced a functional questionnaire, loosely based on the Department of Work and Pensions (UK) (DWP) questionnaires but modified for medical use (see Appendix). This gave me more social and functional capacity information than the tick box DWP form in a standardized way and made it much easier for me to write supporting letters based on reported capacity as well as the findings on a complete physical examination.

As a doctor, one has to accept that over time patients with established ME/CFS may very occasionally develop secondary gain from being ill, which discourages them from adopting health improvement strategies. This too is relatively uncommon, as the majority of patients that I have cared for would give anything or do anything to get even a little bit better. Their burning desire to get better and frustration with the lack of available treatment and support on the NHS often leads them to explore alternative therapies, which may or may not be helpful.

The psychological status of a patient with confirmed ME/CFS is often not conducive to recovery. Repeatedly being told there is nothing wrong with you when you know that there is, is deeply disillusioning and leads to loss of faith in orthodox medicine. The loss of a job leads to severely reduced self-esteem, as does the inability to have or to support a family. Being dependent on others is disheartening and even embarrassing, when for example needing help with personal care. Sufferers' social circle often contracts, as healthy friends cannot understand the illness or make the time for the ME/CFS sufferer. Isolation follows. All of this contributes to secondary depression.

CHAPTER 5

FURTHER READING

Marks DF. The rise and fall of the psychosomatic approach to medically unexplained symptoms, myalgic encephalomyelitis and chronic fatigue syndrome. *Public Health Res.* 2022;1:97–144.

Thoma M, Froehlich L, Hattesohl DB, Quante S, Jason LA, Scheibenbogen C. Why the psychosomatic view on myalgic encephalomyelitis/chronic fatigue syndrome is inconsistent with current evidence and harmful to patients. *Medicina.* 2023;60(1):83. *https://doi.org/10.3390/medicina60010083.*

Vink M, Vink-Niese F. Is it useful to question the recovery behaviour of patients with ME/CFS or Long Covid?. *InHealthcare.* 2022;10(2):392. *https://doi.org/10.3390/healthcare1 0020392*

5.13 Summary and conclusions

It is difficult to make an acceptable summary of all the disparate evidence of abnormalities that have been described in ME/CFS and Long Covid, but the following is an attempt, accepting that it will certainly be proven incorrect as new evidence accumulates. A deep phenotyping study of ME/CFS has concluded that the primary problem is likely to be central and related to the immune response to infection (in the broadest sense). Long Covid almost certainly shares the same pathogenic processes. For a lot of the identified abnormalities, it is hard to know exactly where to place them in the chain of causation.

5.13.1 Triggering of the illness

There may be a genetic predisposition to develop the illness. This includes particular immune response genes (HLA and others, such as FOXP4 in Long Covid).

Significant stress in the preceding 18 months is a risk factor. This may be due to the impact that stress has on the immune system and a reduction in the ability to respond appropriately to infections

It is highly likely that infection is the trigger in a large proportion of cases. Patients with acute-onset illness describe initial features consistent with infection. In most cases, this is likely to be viral and the development of ME/CFS symptoms after acute SARS-CoV2 infection and, to a lesser extent, after the swine flu outbreak and possibly other respiratory viruses, tends to confirm this. Prolonged fatigue has now been reported after the common cold, suggesting that cases of ME/CFS with no apparent trigger may actually be the result of minor or asymptomatic infection with commonly circulating respiratory viruses. However, other viruses may well be involved, including herpesviruses and enteroviruses. Bacterial and protozoal infection are less common triggers.

In many cases the viral infection may be relatively insignificant and will not be sufficient to trigger a request for medical assessment. For the cohort of ME/CFS patients who seem to have a more gradual onset without any obvious initiating infection, the trigger is less clear but could still be a minor and unremarkable viral infection.

5.13.2 Early phase (up to approximately 3 months)

There is little or no information on the early phase of illness in ME/CFS because the diagnosis is never usually made in this time frame and therefore research has not been possible. Occasional patients with severe infections that are later followed by ME/CFS will have come to medical attention, but not enough to generate acute investigations that might illuminate the early phase. To confirm the infective trigger in the majority of patients presenting with ME/CFS would require a huge study of patients who develop infections to identify the specific organisms, who are then followed up for 6 months to identify who develops ME/CFS, which can then be correlated with the identified infections and other biological events.

SARS- CoV2 on the other hand led to a lot of very seriously affected patients and a lot of early-stage research to look at why the illness was so severe. It is clear from these studies that the virus was widely distributed in body tissues, including the brain and the gut and that there was a profoundly damaging acute immunological response, with high levels of pro-inflammatory cytokines, activation of the complement system and thrombotic cascade and the development of autoimmune features in some patients, such as anti-phospholipid antibodies, leading to intracerebral vascular occlusive events. Anamnestic antibodies to CMV and EBV are increased. Other autoantibodies may appear (anti $\beta 2$-adrenoceptors and anti-acetylcholine receptor antibodies?) There is evidence of significant neuroinflammation, with involvement of glial cells. Acute involvement of the brain may well lead to an encephalitic picture. Other quite marked metabolic abnormalities have been described, possibly linked to oxidative stress. Secondary dysfunction of the serotoninergic nervous system may occur due to disruption of the kynurenine pathway, possibly linked to changes in the gut microbiome and virome.

In patients who went on to develop Long Covid, there is clear evidence of damage to the brain and ongoing immunological activity, inappropriate to the stage of infection, suggesting a chronic immune-mediated neuroinflammation, involving microglia. Activation of the thrombotic cascade and complement system suggests the probability of ongoing tissue damage. The normal 'off-switch' for the immunological response to infection seems to be defective. Abnormalities can be detected on MRI scans.

Persistent production of viral proteins in Long Covid suggests a potential mechanism for chronic stimulation of the immune system immune system and secondary chronic inflammatory damage, especially in the brain. It remains to be confirmed whether the same or a similar mechanism is active in ME/CFS.

There may be reactivation of latent viruses (herpesviruses) by the combined effect of acute infection and immunological distraction/dysfunction.

5.13.3 Middle phase (3–12 months)

The ongoing inappropriate immune response and neuroinflammation lead to a range of secondary problems, such as abnormalities of the HPA, autonomic dysfunction (including cardiac dysfunction), mitochondrial abnormalities, bowel abnormalities with dysbiosis, and muscle dysfunction. Persisting neurological dysfunction from the damage caused in the acute and early phases accounts for fatigue, cognitive impairment, and sleep disturbance. By this stage, markers of active viral infection will have disappeared, but there are CSF markers of ongoing brain injury and repair. Microglial dysfunction persists. However, some recent studies have identified the presence of active virus in patients with Long Covid, even at this stage, which would certainly explain ongoing immune activation. Whether the same applies in ME/CFS is uncertain. Chronic illness and chronic inflammation lead to secondary depression.

It has been suggested that overall body response is linked to a 'cells at danger' response as part of an 'integrated stress response (ISR)', leading to shut down of non-essential bodily functions. This is in some respects similar to hibernation or the activation of torpor in rodents and other animals, through a specific hypothalamic nucleus. This response to chronic neuroinflammation shuts down non-essential functions and enables the body to focus on repair (Komaroff & Lipkin, 2021).

5.13.4 Late phase (12 months onwards)

By this stage, there is a significant amount of neurological damage, establishing the chronicity of the illness. There appears to be a skewing of immune responses to a Th2 pattern, which can link with other disorders (mast cell activation, autonomic dysfunction) and a pattern of chronic neuroinflammation. There is no possibility of being able to confirm a triggering infection if patients are seen at this stage, unless CSF or brain biopsies are examined. Secondary changes such as deconditioning become established. Secondary changes to other organ systems also become established, but the evidence for active immunological dysfunction reduces, except in those with severe and persistent symptoms, leaving minor abnormalities of indeterminate significance. By this stage, it is unclear how much of the organ damage, especially to the brain, is likely to be reversible with current treatments. Interestingly, it has been suggested that cyclophosphamide, a potent immunosuppressant, may improve function even in long-term patients, suggesting that there may indeed be some ongoing low-grade immunological damage, even late in the disease process.

When considering trials of treatment, it is necessary to consider which point in the illness trajectory the patient has reached. Therapeutic possibilities will vary according to the stage, with the best chance of influencing the long-term course of the illness being in the early not late stages.

FURTHER READING

Komaroff AL, Lipkin WI. Insights from myalgic encephalomyelitis/chronic fatigue syndrome may help unravel the pathogenesis of postacute COVID-19 syndrome. *Trends Mol Med.* 2021;27(9):895–906. *https://doi.org./10.1016/j.molmed.2021.06.002.*

Walitt B, Singh K, LaMunion SR, et al. Deep phenotyping of post-infectious myalgic encephalomyelitis/chronic fatigue syndrome. *Nat Commun.* 2024;15(1):907. *https://doi. org/10.1038/s41467-024-45107-3.*

CHAPTER 6

What do you tell a patient?

KEY POINTS

- The initial information given to patients has a crucial impact on outcomes.
- Patients need to be encouraged to become 'expert patients'.
- A diagnosis should not be given without a careful history, examination, and at least the minimum set of investigations.
- The diagnosis needs to be presented in a positive way, stressing what can be done to help.
- Follow-up is important to provide answers to new questions, reinforce positive messages, and assist with benefits, school, work, and other issues.
- Females of reproductive years will be anxious about the impact on pregnancy.
- Discussion of boom and bust and how to deal with relapses is very important.

6.1 Introduction

The information given to patients is crucial and may determine the eventual outcome. The information provided is usually dependent on the setting. In the specialist setting, there will be or should be access to a wide range of resources, including experienced doctors and therapists, with supporting paper and electronic resources. Many GPs do not feel comfortable counselling patients, viewing ME/CFS as a rare condition (untrue!) and lacking the time to research suitable resources. Even when regional centres provide information packs and training to primary care, this is often not passed on to patients, the view being that this is the role of the specialist service, despite the evidence that chronic fatigue is a major source of attendance in primary care and that the earlier correct information is provided the better the outcome is likely to be.

It is therefore crucial for patients to be seen promptly in secondary care, so that accurate, up-to-date, and relevant information is given at the earliest possible opportunity. Published evidence confirms that specialist referral centres play a vital role in improving patients' quality of life.

It is also essential to encourage patients to become their own 'expert patient'. This requires a degree of education, so that they develop the skills to evaluate information sourced from the internet and other non-NHS sources. There is a huge amount of information accessible to patients through the internet, but not all of it is correct or helpful.

The appendix gives a useful handout of information sources, through books, internet sites and reputable support organizations for both ME/CFS and Long

Covid, but also for associated conditions. There is an excellent recent review of diagnosis and treatment in the Mayo Clinic proceedings (Bateman et al., 2021), and the NICE Guidelines also summarize best practice (*https://www.nice.org.uk/guidance/ng206*). Guidance is also available for children and adolescents (Rowe et al., 2017). It is however worrying that one-third of children with suspected ME/CFS are not under the care of a specialist service in the UK.

FURTHER READING

Bateman L, Bested AC, Bonilla HF, et al. Myalgic encephalomyelitis/chronic fatigue syndrome: essentials of diagnosis and management. *Mayo Clin Proc.* 2021;**96**(11):2861–78. *https://doi.org/10.1016/j.mayocp.2021.07.004.*

Bayliss K, Riste L, Band R, et al. Implementing resources to support the diagnosis and management of chronic fatigue syndrome/myalgic encephalomyelitis (CFS/ME) in primary care: a qualitative study. *BMC Fam Pract.* 2016;17:66. *https://doi.org/10.1186/s12875-016-0453-8.*

Broughton J, Harris S, Beasant L, et al. Adult patients' experiences of NHS specialist services for chronic fatigue syndrome (CFS/ME): a qualitative study in England. *BMC Health Serv Res.* 2017;17:384. *https://doi.org/10.1186/s12913-017-2337-6.*

Rowe PC, Underhill RA, Friedman KJ, et al. Myalgic encephalomyelitis/chronic fatigue syndrome diagnosis and management in young people: a primer. *Front Pediatr.* 2017;5:121. *https://doi.org/:10.3389/fped.2017.00121.*

Rowe K. Chronic fatigue syndrome/myalgic encephalomyelitis (CFS/ME) in adolescents: practical guidance and management challenges. *Adolesc Health Med Ther.* 2023:13–26. *https://doi.org/10.2147/AHMT.S317314.*

Royston AP, Burge S, Idini I, Brigden A, Pike KC. Management of severe ME/CFS in children and young people in the UK: a British Paediatric Surveillance Unit study. *BMJ Paediatr Open.* 2024;**8**(1):e002436. *https://doi.org/10.1136/bmjpo-2023-002436.*

6.2 At the beginning

The most important part of the initial consultation, once a history and examination has taken place is to find out what the patient thinks might be wrong, what they know or think they know about their condition and in particular to identify any important misbeliefs that will hinder management. This means to begin with listening is more important than speaking. This applies just as much in primary care as in secondary/tertiary care.

I have always been very wary about jumping in with a diagnosis of chronic fatigue until I have satisfied myself that I have excluded all other possibilities, as by the time I retired 47% of my referrals as CFS/ME had other diagnoses confirmed for their fatigue. The other major issue is that almost all patients have been affected by the highly negative views that people have expressed to them, including other healthcare workers. This makes them very wary. It is important to establish a proper rapport with patients, so that they will trust you and believe what you say. This may take several visits. Almost all patients, by the time they have reached a specialist, have experienced inappropriate advice from healthcare workers at some point and so remain suspicious. Most will also have read information for themselves on the internet, which may be both helpful or unhelpful, depending on what they have found! They may bring folders or even boxes of their research.

It is most certainly not helpful to tell them that they just need to get more exercise and they will get better. They will already have tried that and found that it doesn't work (boom and bust). They will strongly resist the notion that 'it is all in their head' or that they are 'depressed' and a course of anti-depressants will make them magically better (they may be slightly happier, but they will still have fatigue!).

It is very important to stress to the patient that having 'normal' test results doesn't automatically equate to the doctor thinking that there is nothing wrong and that therefore the doctor still thinks it is all in the head. The purpose of the tests is to identify simple things that may masquerade as ME/CFS, so normal test results are actually *consistent* with a diagnosis of ME/CFS. Patients will often push for a diagnosis, but because of the difficulties with 'labels' alluded to here, it is wise to decline until there is a certainty that all the information is available, as you will be giving a diagnosis for which, at the moment, there is no magical curative treatment and rather inadequate supportive therapy.

Obviously, once one is happy that the diagnosis IS ME/CFS, then this information must be imparted to the patient. Mostly, they are relieved that, firstly, someone has listened and taken them seriously and, secondly, that they do have the condition that they themselves have concluded that they have. Having a confirmed diagnosis is often the first step on the road to recovery: you can only fight an enemy that has a name!

6.3 When the diagnosis is confirmed

Once the diagnosis is confirmed, it needs to be presented in a positive not negative way. This means focusing on positive things that can be done, rather than just the negative (no treatment, may not get better, etc.). In medicine in general, there is never 'nothing that can be done': it may not be what the patient expects or wants, but there is always something to be done. The majority of my patients, however, were already well aware of the limitations of what could be done, and their main reason for seeking help was for diagnostic validation and help with bureaucratic things like benefits and pensions.

The most crucial thing that the healthcare professional can offer is support and understanding, and this means that someone needs to take responsibility for the long-term, as it is a long-term condition which affects every aspect of life. Here the treatment is 'white-coat medicine'—the doctor is the medicine (even though we do not wear white coats any longer). Voltaire is supposed to have said that the role of the doctor is to amuse the patient until nature effects the cure. 'Support' in this setting means being able to make referrals to people who can provide support, helping with benefits, insurance, and pensions. There are now fewer and fewer people and organizations who can provide such help and support: the government has whittled away support organizations (like Citizens Advice Bureau) and charities struggle with fundraising, even more so following the COVID-19 pandemic. The government makes it harder for ME/CFS patients to claim benefits: the forms are long and complex, and patients with ME/CFS will invariably need help to complete them, but worse, the only medical reports that are acceptable are those from hospital specialists (which the DWP now no longer pay for!). A lot of my support for patients in the longer term revolved around having follow-up appointments specifically to do additional reports for benefits/pensions/insurance. This is even when the patient has been ill for years and is unlikely to make a Lazarus-like recovery (barring any new treatments in the future). Often, I felt that I was doing extra bureaucratic work because the DWP couldn't be trusted to do its job fairly and accurately or just wasn't willing to do it. The experiences of patients with Long Covid are identical.

Once a diagnosis is made, it is important to have up-to-date information about the condition for the patient and their family to take away. Having official information on ME/CFS and Long Covid is very valuable as patients can often experience prejudice within their own wider family, and they need to have something to share with family. I developed over time a handout of resources to deal with most of the questions that came up regularly.

In many areas of England, specific treatment services are available. Although these were set up in 2006-2008 across all of England, many services folded when central ring-fenced fencing was withdrawn. Scotland never really had any widespread services. Many patients come to their clinic appointments with fixed negative views about therapy services because of controversies over graded exercise and cognitive behavioural therapy (CBT). This means that getting buy-in to a referral for therapy can be difficult/impossible. Despite appearances, most therapy services that I worked with had, by the time I retired, moved beyond the proscriptive one-size-fits-all model to a client-centred model. However, many psychologists are still fixated on a biopsychosocial model of causation, which is almost certainly incorrect, and rigid adherence to this often leads to poor engagement or complete disengagement from supportive therapies.

For Long Covid, separate clinics were established, often within departments of respiratory medicine, but as time has passed and with increasing recognition that Long Covid is a form of ME/CFS the services have shared experience and management processes. It certainly does not help to have separate NHS services provide the same care to groups of patients with the same/similar underlying condition.

A lot of the discussion with patients post-diagnosis is therefore about what ME/CFS or Long Covid are and which supportive therapies may help and equally which won't! There are many therapies available outside of the NHS at varying costs to the patient, which are discussed in the chapter on therapies. Clinicians need to take a balanced view: what works for the patient is clearly best for that

CHAPTER 6

patient, bearing in mind that there is a strong placebo response. Patients very reasonably expect their doctors to be familiar with most therapies and offer a reasoned discussion of benefits and risks. At the end of the day, doctors are simply signposts on the journey of life for their patients, so as long as you have provided all the relevant information, it is entirely up to the patient which path they take and the doctors should support this, even if the patient doesn't choose the doctor's own preferred path. The only exception to this rule is where there is doubt about capacity or there is external coercion or where a therapy is frankly dangerous.

Patients are very concerned about the long-term outcomes. It is important to give realistic information on the expected prognosis. This has to be carefully balanced between the unrealistically optimistic and the terminally gloomy. It also needs to take into consideration the often-unbalanced views that can be sourced by the patient. How messages are presented in the early phase post-diagnosis is crucial to long-term outcomes.

FURTHER READING

Horton SM, Poland F, Kale S, et al. Chronic fatigue syndrome/myalgic encephalomyelitis (CFS/ME) in adults: a qualitative study of perspectives from professional practice. *BMC Fam Pract.* 2010;11:89. *https://doi.org/10.1186/1471-2296-11-89.*

6.4 During follow-up

While the NHS would undoubtedly prefer to work on the basis that people with ME/CFS do not have long-term medical follow-up, this is unfair. People with other more 'acceptable' diagnoses get followed up, and ME/CFS and Long Covid are no different to any other long-term conditions with profound impact on health and lifestyle.

The purpose of follow-up is to review with the patient their symptoms and their response to any therapeutic inputs. In particular, one needs to ask about new symptoms. All too often, new symptoms are simply attributed to the ME/CFS or Long Covid when in fact they may be a marker of something new and different. A lot of follow-up is taken up with dealing with schooling, university, employment, benefits, insurance, and pensions. A lot can be more easily (for the patient) done over the telephone unless there are new and suspicious symptoms. It is useful at intervals to get patients to complete a functional questionnaire: this is helpful for preparing reports for benefits, employers, etc. (see Appendix 2).

Follow-up gives the opportunity to reinforce positive changes and to deal with negative and unhelpful behaviours. It also gives the opportunity for discussion of any new therapeutic options and to check whether the patient has started any other treatments without the NHS.

Follow-up is also essential to support the patient with applications for benefits, appeals against benefit decisions, insurance and pension applications, letters to an employer's occupational health department, help with education, and applications for further education. As the DWP has essentially offloaded all the costs of applications, acquiring reports, etc. onto patients, while budget cuts have ensured that access to advice through the Citizens Advice Bureau is restricted, much of this work ends up as *pro bono* work, as patients are in no position to pay for reports, to access help that is their legal right. Help may be available from the ME Association and Action for ME. Preparing accurate reports requires regular contact with patients.

The commonest problems/questions that are reported by patients at follow-up concern how much activity can be undertaken. Activity management is covered in Chapter 8. There is a very fine line between activity adequate to maintain muscle function, postural adaptations, and to enable slow incremental recovery as against overactivity, which will produce boom-and-bust patterns of activity that perpetuate symptoms. Precise advice is difficult and is entirely patient-dependent. The art is in encouraging patients to understand their symptoms and response to activity and adjust their own activity. This should be monitored to ensure that they don't choose to be inappropriately inactive. If they have unavoidable major events, such as a wedding, then it is important to encourage extra rest in the days before and after the event and not be afraid to take rests during the event. Prior explanations to the hosts are important. Specific issues relating to travel are covered in Chapter 11.

It is essential to remind patients that mental activity is as tiring in chronic fatigue as physical activity. There must be a balance between physical and mental activity: more of one means less of the other.

It is important to stress the importance of having a proper daily routine. This should include getting up at a sensible time and getting dressed. Prolonged bed rest is unhelpful. There should be no issue with a nap after lunch provided that this is of short duration and followed by being up until bedtime. Even in the severely incapacitated, it is better to be in a chair than a bed, to maintain the physiological reflexes that support blood pressure in the vertical position.

FURTHER READING

Collin SM, Crawley E. Specialist treatment of chronic fatigue syndrome/ME: a cohort study among adult patients in England. *BMC Health Serv Res.* 2017;17:488. *https://doi.org/10.1186/s12913-017-2437-3.*

6.5 About pregnancy

6.5.1 ME/CFS

A common question that arises in young female patients with ME/CFS relates to pregnancy. There is some limited data to suggest that patients with ME/CFS are more likely to have irregular periods and amenorrhoea or irregular bleeding.

Endometriosis and polycystic ovarian syndrome may be more common, although whether the CFS is the cause of this or merely secondary to these conditions is unclear. It has been suggested that both conditions are linked to mast cell activation, as a response to the Th2 skewing of the immune response seen in ME/CFS and Long Covid. In the 1990s, there was a lot of information circulating in patient fora that pregnancy was definitely bad for patients and would make the illness much worse. In fact, there is no convincing evidence to support this notion, although very little published data about outcomes exists. About 30% of pregnant ME/CFS mothers feel better during pregnancy and 29% feel worse, with the remainder unchanged. Pregnancy has, very rarely, been reported to trigger ME/CFS. Careful management is required during pregnancy to ensure that no other medical conditions of pregnancy develop that would impact on symptoms.

The next question is always about whether delivery should be by elective Caesarean section. ME/CFS is not considered an indication for an elective section. While normal vaginal delivery may be tiring, recovery and the ability to cope with a newborn will be far better without needing to recover from a major surgical procedure on top. Caesarean section should be reserved for the normal indications for this procedure.

It is very important to counsel would-be ME/CFS mums that more of the problems develop from the outcome of pregnancy, that is caring for a newborn and later on an active toddler/child. Prospective mums need to ensure that they have a good support network from their partner, family, and friends. This includes having periods when they can safely rest themselves, with others supervising the child. Breastfeeding is desirable, if possible, but getting the baby to take bottles early (either using expressed milk or formula) will allow others to help with the feeding, especially at night, as the additional sleep disturbance may worsen daytime symptoms of fatigue.

6.5.1 Long Covid

Similar findings have been reported in Long Covid, although there is less data available so far. Management is therefore as for ME/CFS.

FURTHER READING

Pollack B, von Saltza E, McCorkell L, Santos L, Hultman A, Cohen AK, Soares L. Female reproductive health impacts of Long Covid and associated illnesses including ME/CFS, POTS, and connective tissue disorders: a literature review. *Front Rehabil Sci.* 2023;4:1122673. *https://www.frontiersin.org/articles/10.3389/fresc.2023.1122673.*

6.6 About relapses

It is essential that patients with ME/CFS and Long Covid understand from the outset that they may suffer relapses (see Chapter 8.17). These may be triggered by excessive activity ('boom and bust') but also by intercurrent infections, usually viral infections. Activity management ('pacing', see Chapter 8.4) will help reduce the risks of relapses. Careful planning is required where there are major events which the patient recognizes may be beyond their present capabilities, for example, attending a wedding. Planning can include increasing rest before and after the event and taking steps to have extra rest breaks during the event (e.g. have a room planned in which time-out is possible).

For intercurrent infections, most triggering infections will be viral and not amenable to direct treatment. Recognizing symptoms and responding promptly by reducing activity and resting is key. Patients need to understand that although there will be a dip in energy and an increase in symptoms, they will recover faster than previously if they follow the rules for activity management. Trying to soldier on without any reduction in activity will make recovery slower.

The 2021 NICE Guideline contains brief information on managing relapses which is reproduced on the ME Association website, but they also have a more detailed downloadable guide.[1] Patients can be signposted to this.

---

[1] See 2021 NICE Guideline, *Managing flare-ups in symptoms and relapse*—The ME Association, and ME Association, 'Relapses, Exacerbations and Flare-ups', 2023. *https://meassociation.org.uk/wp-content/uplo ads/2025/02/Relapses-exacerbations-and-flare-ups-FEBRUARY-2023.pdf*

CHAPTER 6

CHAPTER 7

Children and young people with ME/CFS or Long Covid

KEY POINTS

- This book is primarily about adults.
- The differential diagnosis of chronic fatigue in children is different.
- Early referral of chronically fatigued children to a consultant paediatrician is essential.
- Managing schooling and peer-group interactions are paramount.

7.1 Diagnosis and management of children

As an adult physician, I was not directly involved with children with ME/CFS, although I would work closely with paediatricians and paediatric therapists. I viewed my remit as starting aged 16 (this was the cut-off for all our other adult clinics). This did, however, mean that I would see young people still in school and thinking about university. ME/CFS and now Long Covid both occur in children of all ages. Children as young as 2 years may be affected. For ME/CFS there is a peak of prevalence between 11 and 19 years. Figures for prevalence vary from 0.75% to 3%. Pre-puberty there appears to be no sex difference but post-puberty the illness is commoner in females than males. Diagnosis of Long Covid in children will be assisted by evidence of the initiating infection with SARS-CoV2. 1-3.5% of children infected with SARS-CoV-2 go on to develop symptoms of Long Covid. Older children seem to be at more risk. There does appear to be more chance of recovery, with only 1% still symptomatic at one year.

The diagnosis of ME/CFS in children is much more difficult, and the differential diagnosis is different compared to adults. Children are not just small adults. NICE Guidance recommends early referral at 4 weeks of children with prolonged fatigue for investigation by an experienced paediatrician.[1] It is concerning that recent evidence suggests that at least one-third of children with ME/CFS are not under the care of a specialist team. Comprehensive assessment is advised to ensure that no other medical illness is present. Symptoms in children tend to be very similar to adults although headaches and stomach pains tend to be more frequent and fatigue may appear to be less of an issue. Disordered sleep is very common. Vasovagal and autonomic problems are common. School absence and/or school

---

[1] See NICE guideline [NG206] (2021), *https://www.nice.org.uk/guidance/ng206*

refusal may be key markers of ME/CFS and this diagnosis should be considered in the management of school refusal.

As noted earlier, the differential diagnosis in children is somewhat different to adults. Consideration must always be given to factitious illness and Munchausen by proxy, although these should be considered carefully and symptoms in children should not be assumed to be factitious unless there is good evidence.

Young people with ME/CFS and Long Covid suffer much more than adults. Being able to interact with their peer group and do the same activities is a crucial part of personal development at this stage of life. ME/CFS and Long Covid can therefore be profoundly isolating (and online chat rooms aren't a substitute). Maintaining young people in school or getting them back into school is often both necessary and difficult. Other fit young people are often not very (at all!) understanding of illness and disability unless they have had other experiences through their own family. This means that a young person with ME/CFS who may be able to go back only part-time and who may need daytime rests may remain excluded, especially if they are unable to do any of the physical activities. It is crucial therefore to get teaching staff on board with the requirements to prevent isolation, bullying, and maintain integration

The most important information to share with the young person and parents is the importance of not taking to bed! Taking to bed guarantees that the normal reflexes that control pulse, blood pressure, and venous return will atrophy rapidly and make the known autonomic dysfunction that is an integral part of ME/CFS and Long Covid worse (see Chapter 5.5). This means that when the person does try and stand, they feel so bad, it reinforces their belief that they need to lie down. Young people often have a better prognosis than adults and therefore it is really important to prevent a lack of activity leading to secondary deconditioning. There are however a small number of severely affected patients who do become bed-bound, and managing this is extremely challenging (see Chapter 8.16). Age-appropriate information is required to reinforce messages. This is available from the national ME/CFS charities (see resources section: Chapter 14.1).

Anxiety and depression are very common in the early stages and should be recognized and managed. Agoraphobia is also common, linked often to fear of how the young person will be perceived by peers. However, the presence of depression and anxiety does not appear to affect the long-term prognosis.

Circadian rhythm disorder is a common cause of fatigue and daytime sleeping in teenagers, especially where there is excessive night-time use of mobile phones/computers and needs to be excluded (see Chapter 4.2).

Supporting regular contact with a few close friends (who 'get' ME/CFS) is essential for maintaining mental well-being. There is always a big issue over the use of wheelchairs and a lot of therapists object to them. My view is that if a wheelchair enables a young person to get out of the house and do things with their parents/friends, then that has to be a positive thing. It does not mean that it is desirable for the person to be in a wheelchair all the time (especially not in the house). Friends can take it in turns to push the wheelchair and when they get to a shop the person can get out and have a short walk around and then get back into the chair (safe refuge). This dramatically expands the range of activities that can be considered. Persuading a young person to use a wheelchair can however be difficult, as they do not want to be seen as even more different! Like any form of disability, the young person with ME/CFS must learn a mindset that they do not care what people think, they are going to use everything that is available to lead as normal a life as possible within the limits their body sets. Over the years I have seen a number of very significant improvements in young people once they started using wheelchairs to get out and about, often to the extent that the recovery speeded up (mainly due to improved mental health) and the wheelchair was gradually downgraded to emergencies only. One affected university student only used her wheelchair for geology field trips (fellow students took turns to push it). It is therefore important, in potentially appropriate cases, to sow the seed about the benefits of wheelchair use early on.

It is important to prevent unwitting collusion of parents with the child's symptoms. Parents need to be encouraged to present a consistently positive but firm approach. This is an extremely difficult balancing act and requires advice to the parents from experienced specialist paediatric therapists.

Another key factor in recovery is the approach of doctors and therapists. Positive support is essential, focusing on what can be done rather than the limitations. Doctors and therapists have an important role in supporting parents and educating schools.

These steps will have a significant impact on prognosis (see Chapter 10.2).

FURTHER READING

Collin SM, Nuevo R, van de Putte EM, et al. Chronic fatigue syndrome (CFS) or myalgic encephalopmyelitis (ME) is different in children compared to adults: a study of UK and Dutch clinical cohorts. *BMJ Open*. 2015;5:e008830. *https://bmjopen.bmj.com/content/bmjopen/5/10/e008830.full.pdf*.

Lopez-Leon S, Wegman-Ostrosky T, Ayuzo del Valle NC, et al. Long Covid in children and adolescents: a systematic review and meta-analyses. *Sci Rep*. 2022;12(1):9950. *https://doi.org/10.1038/s41598-022-13495-5*.

Rowe PC, Underhill RA, Friedman KJ, et al. Myalgic encephaloymelitis/chronic fatigue syndrome diagnosis and management in young people: a primer. *Front Pediatr*. 2017;5:121. *https://www.frontiersin.org/articles/10.3389/fped.2017.00121/full*.

Rowe K. Chronic fatigue syndrome/myalgic encephalomyelitis (CFS/ME) in adolescents: practical guidance and management challenges. *Adolesc Health Med Ther*. 2023;14:13–26. *https://doi.org/10.2147/AHMT.S317314*.

Royston AP, Burge S, Idini I, Brigden A, Pike KC. Management of severe ME/CFS in children and young people in the UK: a British Paediatric Surveillance Unit study. *BMJ Paediatr Open*. 2024;8(1):e002436. *https://doi.org/10.1136/bmjpo-2023-002436*.

What therapies are helpful?

KEY POINTS

- Current advice focuses on activity management and pacing.
- Graded exercise is no longer routinely recommended.
- Cognitive behavioural therapy, mindfulness, and derivatives are useful adjunctive therapies to support patients coping with prolonged debilitating illness but are not curative and may make some patients worse.
- Different therapies may work for individual patients: there is no 'one size fits all'.
- Other therapies with weaker evidence bases are discussed.
- Management of the severely affected is difficult in the UK, as appropriate facilities are very limited.

8.1 Principles of treatment

As, at the time of writing, there are no specific curative therapies, the aim of all treatments should be supportive. Most patients will already have searched Dr Google for information on treatments and may already have some fixed ideas about the benefits or otherwise of certain approaches to treatment. The longer the patient has been ill, the more fixed ideas and attitudes about ME/CFS become. This can be problematic for doctors and therapists and in turn for the patients. The earlier intervention takes place, the better the outcomes will be. This tends to be easier where Long Covid is concerned, because the diagnosis is being recognized much earlier and evidence of COVID-19 infections makes the diagnosis easier. The main focus of treatment for both ME/CFS and Long Covid is about encouraging positive thinking and behaviours and preventing inappropriate behaviours, such as excessive rest in bed, negative thinking, and catastrophizing.

At all stages, therapy needs to be centred around the patient's needs. It must be empathic. The initial stages will be around understanding the patient's current position, their background, and their understanding of their illness. This gives the basis on which to build a professional relationship with the patient based on mutual understanding. The next stage will be to engage in a process of improving understanding of the condition and what can and can't be done to help. All of this takes time. It is important that the healthcare practitioner is fully informed themselves about the condition: nothing ruins the therapeutic relationship faster than the doctor or therapist being found to lack relevant basic knowledge. Therapeutic relationships are built on the trust of the patient that the therapist is well-informed and competent. The advent of the internet means that patients can be at least as knowledgeable as their doctors and therapists, although they may not be able to accurately evaluate all the information that they have discovered. On the other hand, patients do not necessarily expect their doctors to be omniscient. So, it is ok to say that you don't know, as long as that is followed by a commitment to find out and report back.

Where a patient's understanding is radically different from the orthodox view, then the source of these ideas and opinions needs to be explored and alternative views proposed. For this reason, it is important to at least be aware of all types of treatment that are offered, including those outside the NHS and to be able to discuss the risks and benefits of such treatments. In the early stages, in order to maintain the therapeutic relationship, it may be necessary to agree to differ. You can always go back to the issue later as trust develops. Managing chronic fatigue is a long-term process. Concern is frequently raised that therapists (including doctors) should be tougher on patients to avoid colluding with misbeliefs. This is a difficult line to draw: to be effective, it is essential that therapists and doctors retain the confidence of patients. Agreeing to differ is not the same as supporting inappropriate beliefs.

One of the great difficulties for doctors and therapists working in the NHS is in relation to the NICE Guidelines. The initial versions of these were viciously attacked by patient groups for proposing therapies that were felt to make symptoms worse. Subsequent iterations have addressed some but not all of these issues. NHS treatments tend to be offered on a short-term basis only. For a chronic illness of very long or even lifelong duration, these smack of sticking plaster medicine. This will be discussed next in more detail. Guidelines of course are not protocols, although utterances from NICE tend to be treated by NHS managers and bean counters as being requirements. Most therapists who have significant experience of ME/CFS have worked out that the recommended treatment in the NICE Guidelines works for some patients, mainly those who are seen early in their illness. However, other treatment approaches may work better for other patients, especially those who have been ill for years before referral, and so it is vital that healthcare staff keep a reasonably open mind and are preferably familiar with alternative treatment pathways. Doctors and therapists need to be active champions of robust evidence-based therapies.

This brings one to the next major issue and that is the evidence base for any therapy in ME/CFS. The lack of meaningful research during the 1990s and early 2000s means that there is still much work to be done to investigate the best approaches to management. During this period the McEvedy/Beard view that ME/CFS was all psychological and due to hysteria held sway and this seriously impacted the funding of research. Where research trials have been done, the research is often inadequate, with studies that are too small for meaningful statistical analysis and/or lacking proper blinding and placebo controls. Studies in ME/CFS are also plagued by very high response rates to placebos and this means that the number of recruits needs to be much higher and the effect of the treatment much greater before a therapeutic effect can be demonstrated beyond reasonable doubt. Positive results from small insufficiently powered studies that get into the public domain lead to clamour for the treatment to be made available, even when subsequent larger studies fail to show benefit, for example the case of the immunological therapy rituximab (discussed in Chapter 9.8). This places therapists in exceedingly difficult circumstances, as patients assume that refusal to offer the treatment is based on financial grounds and/or the therapists justified scepticism about the illness. This also applies to diagnostic tests, such as the claim that the murine retrovirus XMRV was the cause of ME/CFS, which led to a huge demand to be tested for this virus, even though it was rapidly shown to be incorrect and due to a laboratory error. This strengthens the importance of ensuring an excellent therapeutic relationship with a patient, so that a realistic discussion can take place about potential new therapies, or unproven therapies. All healthcare workers need to ensure that they keep up to date with advances in orthodox and also heterodox thinking, because their patients certainly will be!

Doctors in particular frequently struggle to accept patients' views on alternative therapies. It is inevitable, if orthodox medicine is unable to provide answers and treatments that the patients find useful/acceptable, that they will research heterodox therapies. Simply dismissing the therapies of no value is unhelpful. It is crucial to understand what therapies the patient is following and what their beliefs are about the therapies. It is equally important that the healthcare practitioner is well-informed about the alternative therapies, well enough to have a meaningful discussion with the patient. Where such therapies have been formally evaluated, it may be possible to explain why the therapies may or may not be beneficial. There should not be a presumption that heterodox therapies will be useless. The very high placebo response rate to any therapeutic intervention in chronic fatigue means that, if the patient believes that a therapy will help then they may well derive benefit. The key role of the healthcare practitioner is to be able to discuss the risks of heterodox therapies. Much of the discussion will be about steering patients away from expensive but useless or dangerous therapies.

There is a defining principle in medicine that the doctor should first do no harm, originally attributed to Hippocrates, although it is difficult to confirm that he actually ever said this. However, this does not translate into do nothing! Even in the absence of scientifically proven therapies, the empathic doctor is a therapy in their own right, providing support and guidance.

Largely because of the dominance in the therapeutic debate of psychologists and psychiatrists, most of the therapeutic options offered are based on the concept that ME/CFS is a biopsychosocial illness and therefore psychological therapies will be valuable in treating the illness. As discussed in Chapter 5, knowledge derived from Long Covid and more recent work on ME/CFS is much more suggestive of an underlying organic brain illness, probably autoimmune/inflammatory and triggered by infection either directly or indirectly. Psychological disturbance is therefore likely to be secondary to this, and to the negative attitude of healthcare professionals. Being chronically ill and unable to work and live as normal is profoundly psychologically distressing. Addressing the psychological issues is therefore important but should not be confused with treating the underlying condition. Psychological therapies have a very definite role in helping patients cope with the consequences of chronic illness.

While cognitive behavioural therapy (CBT) is the main recommendation, other psychological therapies are available and often have similarities to CBT. Other psychological therapies may approach the problem from different perspectives. Where one therapy is not effective then it may be worth trying alternatives. All psychological therapies require buy in from the patient (client). Without buy in, the therapy will not work. The referring healthcare worker needs to prepare the ground carefully, explaining what the purpose of the therapy is and especially making it clear that psychological therapies are not 'curative' for ME/CFS or Long Covid but are designed to help the patient cope better.

The most important aspect of therapy is to prevent, as far as possible, deconditioning due to excessive rest. In particular, avoidance of prolonged bed rest is essential. A proportion of the muscular and autonomic dysfunction is due to the illness itself but bedrest does not improve this. This is discussed further below. Again, long delays in reviewing patients in specialized services leads frequently to the patient being substantially deconditioned already by the time they are assessed, which makes managing the fatigue even harder. Explaining about the need to avoid 'boom and bust' early on is essential.

The mental aspect of chronic illness is exceptionally important in determining outcome. There have been many studies that have shown that long-term outcome is related to the mental determination to improve. Psychological input early to reinforce this is therefore a very important aspect of care. Leaving patients without specialist input for months (or years) means that the opportunity to boost coping strategies in a positive way that will influence outcome is missed.

Kim et al. (2020) have carried out an analysis of published trials of therapies for ME/CFS, although quite some trials had to be excluded on the grounds of poor trial design. Overall, more benefit was recorded for non-pharmacological treatments than for drugs, although the advances in understanding the underlying science and pathogenesis may mean that more specific drug therapies are more successful in the future.

At the time of writing, there are no specific drug therapies that are known to be curative. The rapid advances in understanding, in particular the potential role of neuroinflammation in both ME/CFS and Long Covid suggests that more targeted therapies will become available (see Chapter 9). In the meantime, many drugs and heterodox therapies have been tried. Some drugs may well be helpful, but widespread acceptance is hampered by the lack of appropriately powered placebo-controlled trials and dose-ranging studies to confirm benefit. In the absence of any therapies on the NHS, patients may well research and purchase therapies privately. Healthcare professionals need to be aware of these therapies and be able to have an informed discussion with their patients about the potential risks and benefits. The best-known ones are discussed in Chapter 9.

CHAPTER 8

FURTHER READING

Barry PW, Kelley K, Tan T, Finlay I. NICE guideline on ME/CFS: robust advice based on a thorough review of the evidence. *J Neurol Neurosurg Psychiatry*. 2024;**95**(7):671–4. *https://doi.org/10.1136/jnnp-2023-332731*.

Kim DY, Lee JS, Park SY, et al. Systematic review of randomized controlled trials for chronic fatigue syndrome/myalgic encephalomyelitis (CFS/ME). *J Transl Med*. 2020;**18**(7):1. *https://doi.org/10.1186/s12967-019-02196-9*.

Li, J., Zhou, Y., Ma, J. et al. The long-term health outcomes, pathophysiological mechanisms and multidisciplinary management of Long Covid. *Sig Transduct Target Ther*. 2023;**8**:416. *https://doi.org/10.1038/s41392-023-01640-z*.

8.2 General approaches

Early referral to specialist ME/CFS or Long Covid therapy services is essential as early referral is associated with better outcomes. Patients' own pre-consultation research may prejudice them against visiting therapists, usually on the basis that they feel they will be forced into therapies that they have read may be harmful such as graded exercise (GET—see Section 8.5). Careful explanation of the therapists' approaches is required, which in turn requires that referring doctors need to have good liaison with the local teams and to understand exactly what is being offered.

Referral pathways will differ in different geographical locations. Ideally there should be referral pathways from primary care for adults and children, with initial assessment by appropriate adult or paediatric specialists, followed by onward referral to specialist therapists if ME/CFS or Long Covid are confirmed, or further investigation if other conditions are suspected. However, much can be done in primary care to support patients while waiting for assessment.

The first steps in therapy are to explain to the patient, in whom the diagnosis of ME/CFS or Long Covid has been confirmed, the nature of their illness and provide some guidance on the condition from an authoritative source. The patient must be given time to ask questions, as there will most likely be lots of these, sufficient time must be allowed. It may be necessary to spread this introductory part over several visits, as patients with ME/CFS and Long Covid will struggle to think clearly, remember to ask all their questions and then remember what you have said. It is said that patients normally only remember 50% of what their doctor tells them but we have no control over which 50% they will remember! Recall is probably worse in patients with ME/CFS or Long Covid. Long consultations are tiring to patients and the process may need to be spread over several shorter visits. It is important to provide the patient with a written summary of consultations, not only for them but for family members. It is helpful to have printed handouts covering key information. Patient support organizations have downloadable handouts (see Chapter 14.1).

The approach to management, whether in primary or secondary care, needs to be explained. This should include:

1. Nature and causes of the illness, reinforcing the medical, and not psychiatric nature of the illness.
2. The limitations of current treatment.
3. The expected natural history.
4. The importance of self-awareness and self-management (becoming an expert patient).
5. The need to manage activity carefully, avoiding boom-and-bust cycles.
6. The importance of physical exercise within limits (Pacing) to maintain and improve physical function.
7. The importance of mental exercise within limits (pacing!) to maintain and improve cognitive function.
8. The need to balance mental and physical activities each day within the overall energy limits.
9. How to assess activities according to low, medium, and high energy (and how to use diaries).
10. The importance of regular sleep patterns and rests in the middle of the day.
11. The role of psychological therapies to improve coping and secondary depression.
12. The risks and benefits of alternative therapies and OTC medications.
13. How to cope with education/employment/benefits/insurance/pensions.
14. Sources of information and support.
15. Confirmation of follow-up arrangements and referral to other therapists.
16. How to ask for further help.

Secondary depression may become a major feature, particularly in those who have lost a significant amount of their pre-morbid function, self-esteem, and highly paid jobs. This may require very specific counselling and drug treatment, with the clear explanation that this is to treat depression arising as a consequence of the ME/CFS and not to treat the ME/CFS (see next chapter).

Patients often experience sensory intolerance, which is most marked in the more severely affected. This can include intolerance of noises, which not seem particularly loud to healthy people and intolerance of bright light. Intolerance of strong smells can be troublesome, especially household cleaning and air freshen ingredients products, deodorants, perfumes, and aftershaves. There is advice online on alternative unscented cleaning products. Some patients are exquisitely sensitive to the smell and taste of chlorinated water. Small numbers of patients complain of intolerance to electric fields, especially from high voltage overhead power cables.

CHAPTER 8

Specific funded clinics for ME/CFS were established in 2005–2006 in England. The funding was initially directly provided by DHSC, but was later devolved to local levels, whereupon in many cases it largely disappeared! Care models evolved involving clinical psychologists working on biopsychosocial models—the value of which has been questioned more recently as more evidence of the nature of the neuroinflammatory process have come to light. Services are also staffed by physiotherapists and occupational therapists, but in many services therapy staff trained in other modes of therapy and roles became interchangeable. Services in larger centres incorporated a medical element to confirm diagnoses, with some centres insisting on physician screening before referral to therapists. In other services therapists would carry out the screening and only refer cases of concern to physicians. With the increasing awareness of fatigue in other non-ME/CFS illnesses (up to 50% of referrals from primary care), the importance of screening prior to therapy has become more crucial to correct diagnoses. This means that direct referral from primary care to therapists is inadvisable without proper medical screening. Most services have developed strict referral criteria, based on the NICE Guidelines and requiring that the necessary blood tests are carried out before referral and confirmed as normal.

For Long Covid, separate services were set up quickly, now 100 across England, with 13 hubs for children. The total cost as of March 2024 has been £194m. As large numbers of healthcare workers have been affected, the cost to the NHS is substantial and includes sick pay, permanent loss of staff who are unable to return to work (at a time of clinical staff shortage), care costs, and if ligation brought by staff affected, on the grounds that the NHS failed to provide adequate PPE and therefore was negligent in its care of its staff, substantial compensation. Some of these costs are only now being realized and these are on top of the £4–5bn that COVID-19 cost in additional running costs in the first year of the pandemic. It does appear that referrals to Long Covid clinics are now dropping. Newer variants seem less likely to cause Long Covid, and vaccination is largely protective. Unlike ME/CFS, clinics for Long Covid were set up early and have been supported by online resources and a site set up by UCL.[1]

The amount spent directly on care for patients with ME/CFS is far less, although no accurate figure is available, despite the cost to England of the illness being approximately £3.3bn, based on a 0.4% prevalence (2015 figure). Google gives an unverified figure of £542m for 2020 but doesn't give the source or information on what is included in this figure. More accurate figures appear in a 2017 report from Action for ME (*https://www.actionforme.org.uk/uploads/pdfs/2020Health-Counting-the-Cost-Sept-2017.pdf*), which also quotes a total NHS cost of £542m but indicates that only £14m is spent directly on clinical services specific for patients with ME/CFS. Exactly what the remainder of the £542m goes on is unclear, but presumably is on non-specialized services (whose value might

---

[1] See *https://livingwith.health/covid-recovery/* and *https://www.ucl.ac.uk/healthcare-engineering/living-covid-recovery*

CHAPTER 8

be questionable) and other health input. While the DHSC has been consulting about a change to the provision, in the light of medical and therapeutic developments (see: *https://www.gov.uk/government/consultations/improving-the-experien ces-of-people-with-mecfs-interim-delivery-plan* from September 2023), there is as yet no indication as to what if any increase in resources is likely to follow and how it will be distributed. There is a paucity of online resources, but Apps are available via the Apple Store and Google Play but nothing that is endorsed by the NHS.

The devolved nations have largely ignored ME/CFS, with no planned strategy for diagnostic and treatment centres in Scotland, Wales, or Ireland, beyond efforts from individual clinicians. In response to the latest English initiative, the other home nations have simply expressed 'interest'. This means care for patients with ME/CFS in these areas is likely to be very patchy and probably does not meet best practice standards.

8.3 NICE and other guidance

The original NICE Guidelines suggested that patients should be referred for treatment when they had been ill for six months. This was understandable, in the sense that many people have short-term fatigue that resolves, and meeting a definition of 'chronic' fatigue requires that symptoms are of longer duration. It also helped prevent the very limited services being overwhelmed with assessing patients with short-term fatigue and not being able to give sufficient resource to those with longer term symptoms. However, from the patients' perspective this was unhelpful in the extreme, as any potential for early intervention was lost and by the time the patients reached a dedicated service, issues such as loss of jobs, houses, etc. had already taken place, compounding the psychological distress. From a research perspective, opportunities to identify 'hit-and-run' triggering events were also missed. Children were luckier, in that referral earlier was permitted.

For adults, the only therapies recommended were cognitive behaviour therapy and graded exercise. Both caused considerable upset, especially the emphasis on graded exercise. An unsuccessful legal challenge was made against the original guidelines and members of the expert panel that produced them were publicly abused and even received death threats! No other therapies were supported. The biggest cause of upset was the patients' perception that these treatments were viewed by some in the medical profession as curative, whereas in fact most experienced therapists fully recognized that the therapies were only supportive. Graded exercise as an approach has remained under fire, on the grounds that many patients believe that it makes them worse and that pacing is better. The latest iteration of the guidelines, reviewed In 2021, has accepted this.[2] NICE has also produced guidance on managing Long Covid.[3] The current guidance for ME/

---

[2] See NICE guideline [NG206] (2021) *https://www.nice.org.uk/guidance/ng206*
[3] See NICE guideline [NG188] (2020) *https://www.nice.org.uk/guidance/ng188*

CFS has addressed the issue of reducing the time interval for referral from 6 months to 3 months (shorter for children). Despite this, even the latest iteration of the NICE Guidelines has been criticised, prompting a refutation of some of the key criticisms (Barry et al., 2024).

In 2015, the Institute of Medicine in the USA produced a comprehensive review of the diagnosis and management of ME/CFS, while European guidelines have been published in 2021. Both contain much useful information for practitioners in the UK. Guidelines are also available for German-speaking countries (in German).

FURTHER READING

Barry PW, Kelley K, Tan T, Finlay I. NICE guideline on ME/CFS: robust advice based on a thorough review of the evidence. *J Neurol Neurosurg Psychiatry*. 2024;**95**(7):671–4. *https://doi.org/10.1136/jnnp-2023-332731*.

Committee on the Diagnostic Criteria for Myalgic Encephalomyelitis/Chronic Fatigue Syndrome; Board on the Health of Select Populations; Institute of Medicine. *Beyond myalgic encephalomyelitis/chronic fatigue syndrome: redefining an illness*. National Academies Press (US); 2015.

Hoffmann K, Hainzl A, Stingl M, et al. Interdisciplinary, collaborative DA-CH (Germany, Austria and Switzerland) consensus statement concerning the diagnostic and treatment of myalgic encephalomyelitis/chronic fatigue syndrome. *Wiener Klin Wochenschr*. 2024;**136**(Suppl 5):103–23. *https://doi.org/10.1007/s00508-024-02372-y*.

Nacul L, Authier FJ, Scheibenbogen C, et al. European Network on Myalgic Encephalomyelitis/Chronic Fatigue Syndrome (EUROMENE): expert consensus on the diagnosis, service provision, and care of people with ME/CFS in Europe. *Medicina*. 2021;**57**(5):510. *https://doi.org/10.3390/medicina57050510*.

Torjesen I. ME/CFS: Exercise goals should be set by patients and not driven by treatment plan, says NICE. BMJ. 2021;**375**:n2643. *https://doi.org/10.1136/bmj.n2643*.

8.4 Activity management and diaries

Patients need to understand the principles of activity management at an early stage (pacing). This is linked with getting the patient to avoid boom and bust patterns of activity. Teaching patients to categorize activities into high-, medium-, and low-energy activities is essential (this includes not just physical but also mental activities!). Paediatric therapists do this routinely and get the children to fill in daily diaries with different colours for the high/medium/low-energy activities. It can also be very helpful in adults as well. Usually, a 2–4 week period is enough to start with, and this can then be reviewed with the doctor or therapist. The diary should also record how the patient is feeling. At the review, the diary can then help reinforce to the patient how too much high energy activity will correspond to an increase in symptoms 24–48 hours later. Pacing is very helpful in avoiding post-exertional malaise and improving sleep.

Explaining pacing to patients can be difficult. It is the level of activity that a patient can do today and be able to go and do the same level of activity tomorrow and the next day and the next day. If the patient cannot do the same the next day because they are too fatigued, then the level of activity has been too much and needs to be reduced. This must be an iterative learning process for the patient (and also for the doctor/therapist). Only once a stable baseline activity level has been established can the patient look towards changes in activity that will lead to improvement in functional capacity.

The activity baseline will be affected by other internal and external factors. Too much focus is often applied to physical pacing. Mental pacing is just as important. Undertaking a lot of mental activity will reduce the capacity for physical activity and vice versa (see next section). Intercurrent infections will lower the baseline. It can take time and experimentation by both the patient and the therapist to understand the limitations on activity. This is particularly so in patients who have been very physically and/or mentally active before developing chronic fatigue. The baseline will be well below what they are used to doing without a second thought. This presents problems for doctors and therapists, who must rein in the tendency to do far too much too soon and deal with additional depression of mood as reality sinks in.

There is a very useful guide explaining how to pace activity in real-life situations, which goes into this in great detail, which has been published by Ingerbjørd Midsem Dahl (see Chapter 14.1 for details). It is important to recognize that activity management (pacing) MUST be individualized: there is no one-size-fits-all here. Patients also need to understand that is not fixed and will need to be adjusted according to how they feel, what activities must be undertaken, and what activities are planned. It is therefore a fully flexible approach to activity.

Diaries should be a short-term measure. Prolonged use can lead to a negative patient mindset of focusing on what the patient cannot do and how bad their symptoms are, which is unhelpful in the long term. If there are relapses, then another short period of diary keeping can be valuable in identifying areas where changes in behaviour could be made.

Despite the interest in activity management (pacing) for the management of ME/CFS and Long Covid, the actual evidence base confirming benefit is quite limited and the usual problems of small trials with inadequate numbers, lack of placebo groups, etc. have already been highlighted, although meta-analysis of trials is generally favourable.

FURTHER READING

Casson S, Jones MD, Cassar J, et al. The effectiveness of activity pacing interventions for people with chronic fatigue syndrome: a systematic review and meta-analysis. *Disabil Rehabil*. 2023;45(23):3788–802. *https://doi.org/10.1080/09638288.2022.2135776*.

Sanal-Hayes NEM, Mclaughlin M, Hayes LD, et al. A scoping review of 'pacing' for management of myalgic encephalomyelitis/chronic fatigue syndrome (ME/CFS): lessons learned for the Long Covid pandemic. *J Transl Med*. 2023;21:720. *https://doi.org/10.1186/s12967-023-04587-5*.

8.5 Exercise therapy: graded vs. paced

As noted, exercise therapy in chronic fatigue has been the most controversial element of guidelines (PACE Trial, White et al., 2011). The biggest issue has been around 'graded exercise' (GET) which many (most?) patients feel makes them worse. The problem has actually been with the implementation, not so much with the term itself. In the early days patients referred for graded exercise therapy were given utterly unreasonable short-term activity goals, more or less on a one size fits all, which was doomed to fail. The time frames over which 'graded activity' was applied were also inappropriately short. While graded exercise and CBT were the initial recommendations in the first iteration of the NICE Guidelines for managing ME/CFS, patients' experience was very negative, and both patients and patient associations lobbied successfully for GET to be removed from subsequent iterations of the guidelines (NICE guideline NG206), although it took nearly 15 years to achieve this. Subsequent reviews have confirmed the patients' view that it is harmful, at least in the way that it was applied. Even this change has been controversial, with clinicians arguing that it is inappropriate to remove GET and CBT from the guidelines, even though the evidence that supports both GET and CBT is weak and counter-evidence is accumulating.

All the science from sport and exercise medicine over many years, starting from Hanse Selye's general adaptation syndrome (GAS) make it clear that in order to improve physical condition there needs to be regular exercise stress that pushes the body just beyond what it can handle without difficulty. There are three stages. The first stage is an alarm phase when the body recognizes that the exercise stress has increased. This is followed by a resistance phase, when the body has adapted to the increased stress. If the stress is increased too quickly, the body responds with an exhaustion phase. When training athletes, the coach and the athlete have to be able to work out how much physical activity is required to move from the alarm phase to the resistance phase without doing so much that the exhaustion phase is reached.

Physical activity training in ME/CFS and Long Covid is no different to athletic training. The terminology may be different and the target levels very different, but the physiological principles are the same. Pushing too hard or too quickly or both leads to exhaustion, both mental and physical. This is described as 'boom and bust' and almost all patients will recognize this pattern, particularly in the early stages. Post-exertional malaise (PEM) will be increased, along with increased brain fog when too much activity is undertaken. This pattern is usually even worse in those who were physically fit and active before becoming ill, who find it very difficult to adjust their physical activity to a level that is appropriate to their medical condition rather than their previous fitness level. Early explanations about boom and bust are therefore crucial to prevent serial relapses, together with the introduction of the concept of pacing (activity management—see earlier).

The obvious corollary is that every patient needs to have an individualized activity plan (IAP) that is designed for them, just like athletes. There is evidence that this approach is helpful, although why it has taken nearly 20 years for scientists and clinicians to understand that this would be better than one-size-fits-all is beyond my comprehension! This is another example of the compartmentalization of science and medicine, where common knowledge in one area of science is unknown in another!

Patients therefore need to understand that, to improve their physical function, they must be prepared to push gently at their envelope of limitations, while avoiding 'boom and bust'. Just doing the same thing every day will not lead to improvement, although it will prevent deterioration. This is easier said than done. All patients want to get better as fast as possible, so increments in mental and physical exercise need to be very small, and then a new baseline is established before the next small increment. This process is very slow (months, not days or weeks!) and has profound implications for return to school/work.

There is also a strong tendency to focus on physical rehabilitation, while overlooking the fact that this is a brain disorder with reduced cognitive function. A recent study by Greenwood et al. (2014) in Long Covid has confirmed that cognitive, self-care, and physical activities all triggered increases in severity of all symptoms. It can reasonably be assumed that the same occurs in ME/CFS. This means that therapy programmes need to include mental retraining as well as physical retraining. Rehabilitation programmes tend to focus on the physical and overlook the mental. These activities need to include those that stimulate the brain and work on memory. These will be just as tiring as physical activities and therefore each day there needs to be a balance of both physical and mental retraining: boom and bust applies just as much to mental as physical activity. Therapists therefore need to plan both types of activity carefully. Patients need to be aware that on days when they are more active physically, they will have less energy for mental activities and vice versa. I have described it to patients as like being a car with a small petrol tank (or these days a small battery!) which is filled up at night. The patient can use the fuel on whatever activities they like (mental or physical) but once it has gone there won't be any more until the next day. Other have described energy for physical and mental activity like money. You can only spend what you have in your purse. You can borrow from tomorrow's money, but there is an additional cost in terms of 'bust'!

Despite the extensive work on the cognitive deficit in ME/CFS, little research seems to have been done on mental exercises to improve the cognitive problems. Again, this must be tailored to an individual's interests and educational background. Puzzles of all types are valuable; reading is good. However, once the patient has read the same paragraph several times, it is time to stop and rest. There is some interest in using mind–body interventions, but little idea of which interventions add value. More attention is however being paid to the exact defects of cognition found in ME/CFS, which is encouraging (Aoun Sbaiti et al., 2022). There are research studies in progress looking at the use of virtual reality technology to improve mental functioning (Tesarz et al., 2024) and the use of digital apps to help manage symptoms.

CHAPTER 8

There has been and still is a lot of emphasis, especially from patient groups and now in the NICE Guidelines on pacing. Pacing means avoiding boom and bust by limiting activity to a level which does not create exhaustion (see Chapter 5). You will see from what I have said earlier that in order to improve there needs to be an element of pushing at the envelope of activity, so it is difficult for both patient and therapist to identify levels of physical and mental activity that are consistent with pacing but still provide a gentle stimulus to improvement. The patient has to learn to listen to their body and adjust activities accordingly, which can be very difficult. This is where IAPs become very important. These require much more one-to-one work from the therapist and over a longer timeframe. Trying to deal with this in group therapy will not work, apart from explaining the basic principles. Overall meta-analysis, with the usual caveats about trial design, numbers of patients, patient selection, suggests that pacing is effective in managing patient symptoms with ME/CFS. Similar benefit has been described in Long Covid.

FURTHER READING

Aoun Sebaiti M, Hainselin M, Gounden Y, et al. Systematic review and meta-analysis of cognitive impairment in myalgic encephalomyelitis/chronic fatigue syndrome (ME/CFS). *Sci Rep.* 2022;12:2157. *https://doi.org/10.1038/s41598-021-04764-w.*

Bjørkum T, Wang CE. Patients' experience with treatment of chronic fatigue syndrome. *Tidsskrift Nor Laegeforen.* 2009;129(12):1214–16.

Casson S, Jones MD, Cassar J, Kwai N, Lloyd AR, Barry BK, Sandler CX. The effectiveness of activity pacing interventions for people with chronic fatigue syndrome: a systematic review and meta-analysis. *Disabil Rehabil.* 2023;45(23):3788–802. *https://doi.org/10.1080/09638288.2022.2135776.*

Ghali A, Lacombe V, Ravaiau C, et al. The relevance of pacing strategies in managing symptoms of post-COVID-19 syndrome. *J Transl Med.* 2023;21(1):375. *https://doi.org/10.1186/s12967-023-04229-w.*

Greenwood DC, Mansoubi M, Bakerly ND, et al. Physical, cognitive, and social triggers of symptom fluctuations in people living with Long Covid: an intensive longitudinal cohort study. *Lancet Reg Health–Eur.* 2024;46:101082. *https://doi.org/10.1016/j.lanepe.2024.101082.*

Khanpour Ardestani S, Karkhaneh M, Stein E, et al. Systematic review of mind-body interventions to treat myalgic encephalomyelitis/chronic fatigue syndrome. *Medicina.* 2021;57(7):652. *https://doi.org/10.3390/medicina57070652.*

Tesarz J, Lange H, Kirchner M, Görlach A, Eich W, Friederich HC. Efficacy of supervised immersive virtual reality-based training for the treatment of chronic fatigue in post-COVID syndrome: study protocol for a double-blind randomized controlled trial (IFATICO Trial). *Trials.* 2024;25(1):232. *https://doi.org/10.1186/s13063-024-08032-w.*

Twisk FN, Maes M. A review on cognitive behavioural therapy (CBT) and graded exercise therapy (GET) in myalgic encephalomyelitis (ME)/chronic fatigue syndrome (CFS): CBT/GET is not only ineffective and not evidence-based, but also potentially harmful for many patients with ME/CFS. *Neuro Endocrinol Lett.* 2009;30(3):284–99.

CHAPTER 8

Vink M, Vink-Niese A. The updated NICE guidance exposed the serious flaws in CBT and graded exercise therapy trials for ME/CFS. *Healthcare.* 2022;10(5):898. *https://doi.org/ 10.3390/healthcare10050898.*

White PD, Goldsmith KA, Johnson AL, et al. Comparison of adaptive pacing therapy, cognitive behaviour therapy, graded exercise therapy, and specialist medical care for chronic fatigue syndrome (PACE): a randomised trial. *Lancet.* 2011;377(9768):823–36. *https://doi.org/10.1016/S0140-6736(11)60096-2.*

8.6 Rest

The role of rest in recovery from illness is largely misunderstood. When I started in clinical practice, there were still cardiologists who insisted that patients with heart attacks had to have strict bedrest for two weeks. At that time, there was very little that could be done in terms of treatment, but it has become clear not only in cardiology but in most other specialities that prolonged bedrest after acute illness tends to be moderately to severely unhelpful, leading to muscular deconditioning, and complications such as the increased risk of deep venous thrombosis and pulmonary embolism. However, there is some evidence now that muscular deconditioning is not a major factor in perpetuating symptoms of ME/CFS.

Prolonged rest in the horizontal position also leads to gradual loss of the autonomic reflexes that control pulse and blood pressure when humans are standing on two legs. As discussed in the section on the autonomic system, there is evidence that ME/CFS and Long Covid have a direct effect on the autonomic system (see Chapter 5.5), which makes it even more important not to add to this by removing the gravitational drive to activate the autonomic system. The deconditioning of the autonomic system by prolonged recumbency means that attempts to stand will be accompanied by failure of the autonomic responses, leading to a rapid drop in blood pressure and a rise in the pulse rate, accompanied by feelings of dizziness and faintness. This reinforces the feeling that the person should continue to rest recumbent as trying to stand makes them feel worse. I use the analogy of astronauts returning to Earth after a prolonged period of weightlessness in space: they also have deconditioning of the autonomic nervous system and require a prolonged period of readjustment to gravity and vertical posture, to retrain the autonomic reflexes. Experts in autonomic function have shown improvement in CFS patients of all types with a programme of exercises directed at reversing the autonomic problems (Ballentine et al., 2019)

While rest is appropriate in the first days of the acute phase, thereafter it is important to avoid prolonged bed rest. I have always told patients that I don't care how ill they feel they need to be out of bed in the morning, with their legs below their heart. There should always be regular moves from sitting to standing. However, patients with very severe ME/CFS have been shown to have marked reductions in cerebral blood flow even moving from lying to sitting, so caution is required in this group (see Chapter 17). A recumbent rest after lunch is permitted but only as long as it is of limited duration and followed by more rest in a chair, with regular cautious standing.

Patients should be encouraged to do normal things like getting washed and dressed in the morning, even if they need to rest in a chair afterwards. Simple rules about maintaining normal times for waking and bedtime are very important, especially in teenagers and young adults who can very easily slip into sleep reversal (awake all night and asleep all day).

Where medical assessment is delayed and prolonged recumbent bedrest has occurred, autonomic reconditioning is difficult. Exercise programmes specifically to improve autonomic function have been shown to be beneficial. In severe cases, getting an adjustable bed so that the head can be gradually raised and the feet lowered is necessary, before an exercise programme can be started. Provided that this is carried out over a prolonged time period, supervised by an experienced therapist, it can be effective, although up to half the patients may not tolerate the exercise programme (Kujawski et al., 2021).

A study from 2023 (Moore et al., 2023) has shown quite clearly that patients with ME/CFS take up to two weeks to recover from cardiopulmonary exercise testing, compared to 2 days for normal subjects, which confirms patients' experiences of post-exertional malaise. Overall, the best plan is to avoid prolonged bed rest from the start rather than dealing with the consequences later.

Management of sleep disturbance is difficult, but correct management of activity and rest, with pacing and avoidance of boom and bust will improve the quality of sleep. Increasing sleep disturbance is usually a marker of overactivity. To maintain the normal pattern of sleep/wakefulness, prolonged daytime sleeping should be avoided. The normal circadian rhythm runs on a 24-hour cycle with a dip in wakefulness in the middle of the day, but not to the same extent as at night. Many bodily functions, including the immune system have a 12-hour cycle imposed on the normal 24-hour cycle. Thus, having a short sleep after lunch is not abnormal, hence the siesta in Mediterranean countries. Indeed, there is some evidence that suggests having an after-lunch sleep may reduce risks of dementia! For fatigued patients it is important that any afternoon sleep is short and followed by a return to activities consistent with pacing.

There is evidence of circadian rhythm disturbance in both ME/CFS and Long Covid, as part of the illness and not just a response to overactivity, although rigorous studies where all external factors known to affect the circadian rhythm have been controlled are lacking. Disturbance of the circadian rhythm may be attributed to the alteration of cytokine levels, especially TGF-β, although resistin (produced by adipocytes) may also be involved. Low vitamin D, in conjunction with reduced light exposure may also contribute, another reason to check vitamin D, especially in housebound patients.

As discussed in Chapter 4, the differential diagnosis of ME/CFS includes a range of sleep disorders and it is important that any disturbance of sleep is considered in the light of this differential diagnosis.

CHAPTER 8

FURTHER READING

Ballantine R, Strassheim V, Newton J. Gravity-induced exercise intervention in an individual with chronic fatigue syndrome/myalgic encephalomyeltis and postural tachycardia syndrome: a case report. *Int J Ther Rehabil*. 2019;26(5):1–3. *https://doi.org/10.12968/ijtr.2016.0035*.

Bazelmans E, Bleijenberg G, van der Meer JW, Folgering H. Is physical deconditioning a perpetuating factor in chronic fatigue syndrome? A controlled study on maximal exercise performance and relations with fatigue, impairment and physical activity. *Psychol Med*. 2001;31(1):107–14. *https://doi.org/10.1017/S0033291799003189*.

Kujawski S, Cossington J, Słomko J, et al. Relationship between cardiopulmonary, mitochondrial and autonomic nervous system function improvement after an individualised activity programme upon chronic fatigue syndrome patients. *J Clin Med*. 2021;10(7):1542. *https://doi.org/10.3390/jcm10071542*.

Lu S, Wei F, Li G. The evolution of the concept of stress and the framework of the stress system. *Cell Stress*. 2021;5(6):76. *https://doi.org/10.15698/cst2021.06.250*.

McCarthy MJ. Circadian rhythm disruption in myalgic encephalomyelitis/chronic fatigue syndrome: implications for the post-acute sequelae of COVID-19. *Brain Behav Immun Health*. 2022;20:100412. *https://doi.org/10.1016/j.bbih.2022.100412*.

Moore GE, Keller BA, Stevens J, et al. Recovery from exercise in persons with myalgic encephalomyelitis/chronic fatigue syndrome (ME/CFS). *Medicina*. 2023;59(3):571. *https://doi.org/10.3390/medicina59030571*.

van Campen CL, Visser FC. Comparison of the degree of deconditioning in myalgic encephalomyelitis/chronic fatigue syndrome (ME/CFS) patients with and without orthostatic intolerance. *Med Res Arch*. 2022;10(6). *https://doi.org/10.18103/mra.v10i6.2858*.

8.7 Cognitive behavioural therapy

Cognitive behavioural therapy is a well-established psychological therapy which has been shown to be valuable in managing depression, anxiety, phobias, and other mental illnesses. It is based on the concept that problems are caused by unhelpful or faulty thinking leading to unhelpful learned behaviour, particularly catastrophization, where the patient focuses intently on the potential harm that they believe will accrue from active rehabilitation. The therapy is therefore designed to change the person's thinking by getting them to understand how their thinking is leading to unhelpful responses and then training them to think differently and develop better problem-solving skills. In a nutshell it aims to replace unhelpful negative thinking with positive helpful thinking, which can include facing fears and learning to control emotions. CBT is designed as a short-term intervention, usually involving a fixed number of sessions.

It is therefore apparent that, while CBT may help patients cope with chronic illness better, it is unlikely to have a profound effect on the underlying pathology and therefore cannot be considered a curative therapy. That is unless you believe, erroneously, that ME/CFS is purely a psychological illness, which the more recent scientific advances discussed in Chapter 5 suggest is unlikely. Focusing on CBT enables the NHS to offer short, fixed-term therapy, while avoiding providing long-term support, which is actually what is required.

Because many patients come to specialist services with preconceived views about psychological therapies, based on information on the internet and social media, the specialist referring the doctor, as well as the GP and therapists all need to sing from the same hymn sheet about the reasons for the therapy and the likely benefits. They will need to sell the therapy to the patient. Like all psychological interventions, it will only work if there is good buy-in from the patient. Even in the best hands, many patients do not feel they have benefitted from CBT, but that may depend on the initial expectations.

Most recent reviews and meta-analyses of CBT in ME/CFS have been less enthusiastic about the benefits and have drawn attention to methodological flaws in the early trials demonstrating benefit. Analysis has been hampered by the polarized views about whether graded exercise therapy and CBT cause harm. Internal audits by therapy teams often show that while severity scores do not change much after input including CBT, patients feel better. There is no compelling evidence that CBT causes harm, although its benefits may be limited. The most recent iteration of the NICE Guidelines (NICE guideline NG206) makes no specific mention of either CBT or GET. The role of CBT in Long Covid is equally unclear, with benefit shown in some studies but limited or no benefit shown in other studies. Benefit seems most likely to be reported in milder cases, with a reduction in fatigue, persisting for at least 6 months. Up till now, reported trials have been relatively small and not placebo controlled.

Other psychologically based therapies are also available and may be used and preferred by patients. Some of these are discussed next. Uptake of alternatives into NHS practice has been slow/non-existent and this obviously hampers effective comparative research.

FURTHER READING

Ebell MH. Cognitive behavior therapy effective in patients with fatigue associated with Long Covid. *Am Fam Physician.* 2024;109(3):283B–C.

Huth D, Bräscher AK, Tholl S, et al. Cognitive-behavioral therapy for patients with post-COVID-19 condition (CBT-PCC): a feasibility trial. *Psychol Med.* 2023:1–1. *https://doi.org/10.1017/s0033291723002921.*

Kuut TA, Buffart LM, Braamse AM, et al. Does the effect of cognitive behavior therapy for chronic fatigue syndrome (ME/CFS) vary by patient characteristics? A systematic review and individual patient data meta-analysis. *Psychol Med.* 2023;54(3):447–56. *https://doi.org/10.1017/S0033291723003148.*

Kuut TA, Müller F, Csorba I, et al. Efficacy of cognitive-behavioral therapy targeting severe fatigue following coronavirus disease 2019: results of a randomized controlled trial. *Clin Infect Dis.* 2023;77(5):687–95. *https://doi.org/10.1093/cid/ciad257.*

CHAPTER 8

Vink M, Vink-Niese A. The updated NICE guidance exposed the serious flaws in CBT and graded exercise therapy trials for ME/CFS. *Healthcare*. 2022;10:898. *https://doi.org/10.3390/healthcare10050898*.

8.8 Mindfulness

Mindfulness, in the context of medicine, was introduced by Jon Kabat-Zinn. He was working as a psychologist at the University of Massachusetts Medical Center but was also a practising Buddhist who meditated regularly. He developed mindfulness based on meditative principles initially in response to a request from the pain management team to develop a programme to support patients with chronic pain. Gradually, his programme of mindful meditation expanded to take in all sorts of other chronic medical problems, including reducing apparently drug-resistant hypertension. The benefits were marked. He has published many papers on scientific evaluations of the technique in different medical and psychiatric conditions and a number of self-help books. Mindfulness is based on ancient meditation traditions, which are still used today.

Key to mindfulness is learning to live in the moment and being more aware of that moment through feeling and understanding the body and its surroundings, with acceptance but without judgement. This involves being more aware of the body through a body scan. Since Kabat-Zinn introduced it into medicine, its use has become widespread and it has evolved. One thing that Kabat-Zinn has been firm about is that mindfulness is not a 'cure' for anything but is a better way of coping with life. In fact, he gets very annoyed by people claiming that mindfulness will cure conditions!

Mindfulness has permeated into many other therapeutic approaches. As is the way with most psychological approaches, it has grown like a tree, with new branches, not all of which are true to the origins and not all of which understand the ancient principles that underlie mindfulness, so it is useful to go back to Kabat-Zinn's original approach. Mindfulness can be combined with CBT. Many books on the application of mindfulness to ME/CFS have been published. However, mindfulness is something that is very hard to learn for yourself as trying to follow instructions in a book while trying to achieve a mindful state of mind is virtually impossible as the concentration required to read breaks up the mindful state. It is therefore much better for patients to find a competent instructor familiar with ME/CFS or Long Covid.

A particular variant of mindfulness, used in chronic pain and other chronic conditions and occasionally in ME/CFS is acceptance and commitment therapy (ACT). It is considered to be a 'third wave' behavioural therapy, along with other mindfulness-based therapies such as dialectical behaviour therapy (DBT), mindfulness-based CBT (MCBT) and mindfulness-based stress reduction (MBSR). Its aim is to encourage acceptance of symptoms and to stop individuals fighting against their symptoms, which it believes makes the illness worse. It does not aim to reduce symptoms directly but to reduce the impact of the symptoms.

My experience suggests that mindfulness and its variants are more beneficial than CBT alone in ME/CFS, as they lead to a more profound and long-term change in thinking and behaviour. Unfortunately, much of the published evidence suffers from the usual problems of research in ME/CFS. A meta-analysis identified problems of small studies, heterogeneous patient selection, and lack of control groups. Overall, there is a trend to benefit.

Mindfulness has been used acutely during the coronavirus pandemic to help stressed staff, with a number of publications. Evidence for benefit in Long Covid is yet to emerge, although benefit was derived from a very short-term intervention in a small number of patients.

FURTHER READING

Dayes JE. Myalgic encephalomyelitis/chronic fatigue syndrome: a discussion of cognitive behavioural therapy, mindfulness, and mindfulness-based cognitive therapy. *Counsell Psychol Rev.* 2011;**26**(2):70–5.

Hausswirth C, Schmit C, Rougier Y, Coste A. Positive impacts of a four-week neuro-meditation program on cognitive function in post-acute sequelae of COVID-19 patients: a randomized controlled trial. *Int J Environ Res Public Health.* 2023;**20**(2):1361. *https://doi.org/10.3390/ijerph20021361.*

Khanpour Ardestani S, Karkhaneh M, Stein E, et al. Systematic review of mind-body interventions to treat myalgic encephalomyelitis/chronic fatigue syndrome. *Medicina.* 2021;**57**:652. *https://doi.org/10.3390/medicina57070652.*

8.9 Breathworks

Breathworks is another offshoot of mindfulness, focusing on 'loving kindness'. It is actually a registered company offering courses and training for practitioners. It is very similar to mindfulness-based CBT. The founders in the UK received training from Jon Kabat-Zinn and one of the founders is an ordained practising Buddhist. Programmes were initially designed for those with chronic pain, but it has been used by some NHS ME/CFS therapists. It is clearly helpful in this setting, although formal controlled trials are lacking. A recent book aimed at therapists covers this area (McKechnie, 2023).

FURTHER READING

McKechnie F. *Mindfulness-based therapy for managing fatigue: supporting people with ME/CFS, fibromyalgia and Long Covid.* Jessica Kingsley Publishers; 2023.

8.10 Lightning Process and neurolinguistic programming

Neurolinguistic programming has been described as a pseudoscience, because the underlying concepts do not seem to correlate well with current neurological science and the fact that, as a psychotherapy, there is little objective evidence of clinical benefit. It has been mainly used as part of leadership training. There have been multiple legal cases over the rights to use NLP between the co-founders and other parties. There are no certifying bodies and anyone can claim to be an NLP practitioner, which makes it very hard for the general public to choose reputable therapists.

The Lightning Process, pioneered by an osteopath Phil Parker, in the UK, is based to some extent on NLP principles with osteopathy. It is a copyrighted programme. This is provided as a three-day intensive course, although published details tend to be scanty. The course is very intensive, which seems counterintuitive for a group of patients who are easily exhausted. It is supposed to work to counteract negative thoughts and affirm positive thoughts. Patients must be committed to making changes in their life (i.e. want to get better). We know that the outcomes for those who take a positive attitude are more likely to improve, whatever treatment is offered. It is expensive. The NHS and NICE do not support its use, although a small trial in children with ME/CFS did show benefit. However, the trial has been widely criticised. There is a complete lack of acceptable adult clinical trials in ME/CFS, so it is impossible to say whether the benefit in children is replicated in adults. A study in Norway claimed that it was strongly associated with the worsening of ME/CFS symptoms (Wold et al., 2024), and there have also been reports of suicides in patients who have 'failed' the therapy. Phil Parker himself has received death threats. Advertising Standards Agencies in both the UK and Norway have ruled that the Lightning Process advertising that it could cure ME/CFS is misleading see for example https://meassociation.org.uk/2017/11/advertising-standards-authority-ruling-on-me-association-complaint-re-kathy-kent-and-the-lightning-process-15-november-2017/.

Over the years I have seen a small number of adult patients including some young adults who have paid for the treatment. One clearly had no benefit, while the remainder (about four or five) did benefit, in several cases substantially, although two later relapsed. One of those who relapsed had no benefit from a further course. None experienced any obvious adverse effects. This is of course not a scientific study! Bearing in mind the placebo response rate in ME/CFS, these results could simply have occurred by chance. Phil Parker has published the application of the Lightning Process to Long Covid.

Until there are large-scale clinical trials with appropriate placebo groups that demonstrate meaningful clinical benefit, the jury remains out on this therapy.

FURTHER READING

Burns S, Finch F, Parker P, Nollett C. The novel application of the lightning process to treat Long Covid in primary care. *J Exp Psychother*. 2021;24(4):96.

Crawley E, Mills N, Hollingworth W, et al. Comparing specialist medical care with specialist medical care plus the Lightning Process® for chronic fatigue syndrome or myalgic encephalomyelitis (CFS/ME): study protocol for a randomised controlled trial (SMILE Trial). *Trials*. 2013;14:444. https://doi.org/10.1186/1745-6215-14-444.

Crawley EM, Gaunt DM, Garfield K, et al. Clinical and cost-effectiveness of the Lightning Process in addition to specialist medical care for paediatric chronic fatigue syndrome:

randomised controlled trial. *Arch Dis Child*. 2018;103(2):155–64. *https://doi.org/ 10.1136/archdischild-2017-313375*.

Wold BK, Tveito K, Angelsen A, et al. Symptom-based survey diagnoses may serve to identify more homogenous sub-groups of fatigue and postviral diseases. *Fatigue*. 2024;12:261–77. *https://doi.org/10.1080/21641846.2024.2370209*.

8.11 Gupta technique

The basic hypothesis underlying the Gupta technique is that illnesses such as ME/ CFS are a brain overreaction that triggers an unconscious 'protective mode' in the limbic system, related to the amygdala. The technique therefore aims to reduce this overprotective mode by retraining the brain in a holistic way and interrupting the brain circuits involved, particularly those involving the amygdala and the insula. These areas are associated with severe emotions such as fear and rage. It has been used successfully in Long Covid, although proper randomized clinical trials in ME/CFS are lacking. The results in Long Covid suggested a response rate of around 47%. It is also said to be beneficial in fibromyalgia.

Like all psychological therapies tried in ME/CFS it is likely that there will be a high placebo response rate. If Long Covid is anything to go by, the reported 47% improvement is about the level of placebo response seen in some ME/CFS clinical trials, so it will be difficult to prove benefit without very large trials (preferably with a sham treatment arm). We know from other therapies that the technique may not be useful for all patients.

FURTHER READING

Toussaint LL, Bratty AJ. Amygdala and insula retraining (AIR) significantly reduces fatigue and increases energy in people with Long Covid. *Evid-Based Complement Alternat Med*. 2023;2023:7068326. *https://doi.org/10.1155/2023/7068326*.

8.12 Perrin technique

The Perrin technique is a physical therapy, based on improving lymphatic drainage and cranial osteopathy, which was developed by a UK osteopath, Raymond Perrin. He developed his own set of cardinal signs, which do not map to established diagnostic criteria, but which he believes enable practitioners to gauge the severity of symptoms and response to treatment. He believes that toxins accumulate in patients due to impaired cranial lymphatic drainage, which interferes with the autonomic nervous system and leads to a build-up of choline in the brain, which causes symptoms. Curiously, choline supplements have a long history of being used as a *treatment* for ME/CFS by some private practitioners! He has published a guide to the use of his technique in ME/CFS, now in its second edition. However, despite its popularity in the UK with ME/CFS sufferers, there is no robust clinical evidence of benefit and the underlying theory is dubious. No obvious harm has been reported. Perrin has also reported on its use in Long Covid.

FURTHER READING

Heald AH, Perrin R, Walther A, et al. Reducing fatigue-related symptoms in Long COVID-19: a preliminary report of a lymphatic drainage intervention. *Cardiovasc Endocrinol Metab.* 2022;11(2):e0261. *https://doi.org/10.1097/xce.0000000000000253.*

Perrin R. *The Perrin technique 2nd edition. How to diagnose and treat chronic fatigue syndrome/ME and fibromyalgia via the lymphatic drainage of the brain.* Hammersmith Health Books; 2021.

Perrin RN. Lymphatic drainage of the neuraxis in chronic fatigue syndrome: a hypothetical model for the cranial rhythmic impulse. *J Osteopath Assoc.* 2007;107(6):218–24.

8.13 Diet

A huge amount has been written about diet and ME/CFS and almost all known diets have been tried, without any convincing evidence that any specific dietary manipulation has a major effect on the majority of patients. A recent small study in Australia found that a cohort of ME/CFS patients were self-managing with a wide range of nutritional modifications and supplements but failed to show that any modifications correlated with improvement. At the research level there is interest in the potential of alterations in the gut microbiome to cause or contribute to disease (dysbiosis)—see Chapter 5.10. It is increasingly clear that there are direct links between the gut and the brain, as well as between the gut and the immune system. Other suggested causes of problems are the production of D-lactic acid in the gut which it is thought may contribute to neurological problems, increased bowel permeability, and alterations in kynurenine metabolism, with abnormalities of the enzyme indole-2,3-dioxygenase, leading to changes in tryptophan metabolism. However, at present, none of the mechanistic research is advanced enough to be able to pronounce on a definitive dietary strategy for ME/CFS or Long Covid.

As part of the evaluation of a patient with ME/CFS it is essential to ensure that there is no evidence of nutritional deficiency, especially if the person is on any kind of restrictive diet. Blood tests should be undertaken to assess iron status, as well as B_{12} and folate. In Northern latitudes it is also essential to measure vitamin D, as deficiency is increasingly common the further north a person lives (see Chapter 3.3).

Exclusion of coeliac disease should be part of the screening and should be undertaken with the person on a gluten-containing diet. Many people with ME/CFS feel better on wheat-free diets, although there is no obvious scientific basis for this. A wheat-free diet is not the same as a gluten-free diet.

Another favourite is the anti-candida diet, even though there is no evidence that candida plays any role in causation on maintenance of ME/CFS. The diet involves avoiding high-sugar foods and yeast-containing foods such as breads and fermented products (beer). The diet is not harmful and almost certainly will benefit irritable bowel symptoms, which are common in ME/CFS and Long Covid.

As almost all patients with ME/CFS have symptoms of irritable bowel syndrome, diets used to treat this condition may be required. Patients with IBS symptoms may respond well to different types of diet, for example, low fibre or high fibre, avoiding reprocessed starchy foods (recooked bread, potato, etc.), avoiding wheat, or the FODMAP diet (fermentable oligosaccharides, disaccharides, monosaccharides, and polyols (which are sugar alcohols)).

Anti-inflammatory and fatigue-reduction diets may also be tried. These tend to have been tried in other disorders and in cancer. They tend to be healthy diets with plenty of fresh green and yellow/orange fruits and vegetables, nuts and seeds, whole grains and fish, and fish oil. It tends to be high in fibre and low in fat and may not suit some patients with significant irritable bowel syndrome. However, the diets are healthy.

Vegan (plant-based) diets may also be tried. These may be deficient in certain essential amino acids and in certain vitamins and minerals, so specific advice on how to avoid these deficiencies is required. People on vegan diets say that they have more energy. Fatigue and fibromyalgia pain may be improved. The ideal vegan diet is one that avoids highly processed alternatives to meat. There is some evidence that long-term health can be adversely affected by vegan diets which contain high levels of highly processed vegan foods.

Ideally, patients should be encouraged to have a healthy diet with a broad range of foodstuffs, to maintain a balanced nutritional status. This includes having an appropriate balance of carbohydrate, fat, and protein, appropriate to activity levels. The possibility of eating disorders needs to be considered. Review by a dietician may be required to evaluate nutritional input.

Vitamin and mineral supplements should not be required unless there is clear evidence of deficiency. Any significant modification to the diet should be undertaken with input from a state-registered dietician (not a nutritionist). There is no evidence that mega-doses of vitamins are helpful and excess intake of some, such as vitamin C, which can cause kidney stones, or iron, which can damage the liver, can be harmful to health. Vitamin C, together with vitamin E and α-lipoic acid are thought to be anti-oxidants. Supplementation has been reported to improve some symptoms, such as fatigue, sleep, and headaches.

Supplemental vitamin B_{12} has been suggested but is not recommended unless there is clear evidence of deficiency and/or the presence of gastric parietal cell antibodies, which are linked with pernicious anaemia and vitamin B_{12} deficiency. In the absence of evidence for pernicious anaemia or terminal lineal disease (where vitamin B_{12} is absorbed), oral supplements only can be supported. Intramuscular B_{12} is only justified in conditions where absorption is impaired. There have been suggestions, derived from studies of metabolites associated with B_{12} that patients with ME/CFS have a functional deficiency in B_{12} that can be ameliorated with i.m. B_{12}. Only small trials have been carried out and not all patients respond.

CHAPTER 8

A confounding factor is that vitamin B_{12} injections tend to induce a general sense of well-being even in B_{12}-replete individuals. No side effects appear to be reported from having very high levels of vitamin B_{12}, despite the fact that it is stored in the liver.

Other nutritional supplements for which there is some (limited!) evidence are acetyl-L-carnitine and essential fatty acids (gamma-linoleic acid from evening primrose oil and eicosapentanoic acid from fish oil). None of the trials have been large or have included placebos, but benefit appears to have been reported in ME/CFS patients. None of these compounds appear harmful and all are available over the counter.

D-ribose (a component of ATP) has been used to improve ATP levels. It is claimed that supplementation improves energy and sleep and reduces pain. However, the trials have been small and uncontrolled.

Extracts of Gingko biloba are reported to have antioxidant properties. It is thought to improve cognitive function and is marketed as such over the counter. Trials using it in combination with cistanche (a Chinese herbal medication) have suggested it improves fatigue, post-exertional malaise, and unrefreshing sleep.

There is some evidence that levels of anti-oxidants are low in ME/CFS, and some practitioners recommend supplementation with anti-oxidants (vitamin C, vitamin E, selenium). However, formal double-blind placebo-controlled trials have not been conducted. In exercise medicine, there are similar findings, and it was hypothesized that supplementation would lead to faster recovery and muscle repair. However, trials have shown that there is minimal benefit and that in fact high doses of antioxidants may actually impair immune function and repair. As high-dose vitamin C can lead to excessive oxalate production and kidney stones, caution should be observed in high-dose vitamin C use.

Probiotics are often tried, although evidence for benefit is scanty. Our use of probiotics is primitive, focusing on 2–3 bacteria, whereas the gut microbiome may contain upwards of a thousand species of bacteria, many of which are known only by their genetic signatures. It has been suggested that faecal transplants from healthy individuals may be the only way to recreate a 'normal' gut microbiome in a sick patient. The whole issue of which bacteria are actually required for a healthy gut is still a work in progress. Any change to the base diet is known to significantly alter bacterial flora and while there are suspicions that presence or absence of certain types of bacteria may be associated with disease, it is not yet proven whether these changes are cause or effect. It has been suggested that the use of probiotics should reduce the production of D-lactate, which has been associated with symptoms. While some studies have shown an improvement in symptoms with probiotics, no changes in D-lactate were noted.

Patients will often experiment with other health food supplements, sometimes with benefit and sometimes not. Provided that there is no evidence of health risk, then there can be no objection. Some supplements have been associated with severe side effects, especially in the liver (black cohosh). The availability of supplements in a health food shop is no guarantee of safety or lack of side effects.

Equally for almost all supplements, the actual level of active ingredients may vary from one brand to another and may not correlate with that stated on the label. As they are classified as food supplements, there is little or no oversight. Patients should be advised to avoid spending large sums of money on supplements unless there is convincing evidence of benefit. It is wise to advise patients, if they wish to try supplements, to have a 1–2 month trial and then a period off to see whether they can truly identify a benefit.

If the patient is taking prescribed medication, then they need to check for interactions with herbal remedies and other supplements. For example, prescribed SSRIs can interact with a range of OTC supplements and foods, causing serotonin syndrome.

Patients should be advised to limit alcohol and caffeine consumption, as both make symptoms worse. Sensory intolerance in ME/CFS and Long Covid will often have an impact on the sense of smell and taste, and this can have an impact on diet, and in some cases lead to inadequate consumption of protein and carbohydrate.

FURTHER READING

Seton KA, Espejo-Oltra JA, Giménez-Orenga K, Haagmans R, Ramadan DJ, Mehlsen J. Advancing research and treatment: an overview of clinical trials in myalgic encephalomyelitis/chronic fatigue syndrome (ME/CFS) and future perspectives. *J Clin Med*. 2024;13(2):325. *https://doi.org/10.3390/jcm13020325*.

Weigel B, Eaton-Fitch N, Passmore R, Cabanas H, Staines D, Marshall-Gradisnik S. A preliminary investigation of nutritional intake and supplement use in Australians with myalgic encephalomyelitis/chronic fatigue syndrome and the implications on health-related quality of life. *Food Nutr Res*. 2021;65. *https://doi.org/10.29219/fnr.v65.5730*.

8.14 Cryotherapy

Cryotherapy has been shown in animal and human experiments to improve immune function and reduce inflammation. Wim Hof is a particular exponent of ice-cold immersion with meditation, and some of his trainees have been investigated. There are suggestions that it may help fibromyalgia and that the combination of cryotherapy with static stretching may benefit patients with ME/CFS, through an effect on the autonomic nervous syndrome. How widely this is applicable is unknown.

FURTHER READING

Kujawski S, Słomko J, Godlewska BR, et al. Combination of whole body cryotherapy with static stretching exercises reduces fatigue and improves functioning of the autonomic nervous system in chronic fatigue syndrome. *J Transl Med*. 2022;20:273. *https://doi.org/10.1186/s12967-022-03460-1*.

8.15 Managing disordered sleep

Little is written specifically about managing disordered sleep in ME/CFS and Long Covid. Patients with both conditions report disturbed and unrefreshing sleep, and this forms part of the diagnostic criteria. From the practical perspective, the level of disordered sleep is linked to the severity of the other symptoms, such as post-exertional malaise, fatigue, and cognitive disturbance. It is quite clear that boom phases of overactivity lead to an increase in sleep disturbance and that this in turn contributes to the increase in other symptoms in the bust phase. There is some evidence to support a primary disruption of circadian rhythms in both ME/CFS and Long Covid. In young people specifically it is crucial to exclude circadian rhythm disorder as the primary diagnosis, and in older people other primary sleep disorders (see Chapter 4.2). General management of activity should improve sleep quality. Avoidance of caffeine and alcohol in the evening is important. Likewise, mobile phones, computers, and televisions should not be used in bedrooms, as they emit blue light that prevents the onset of sleep. Drug therapy for sleep is discussed in Chapter 9.4.

FURTHER READING

McCarthy MJ. Circadian rhythm disruption in myalgic encephalomyelitis/chronic fatigue syndrome: implications for the post-acute sequelae of COVID-19. *Brain Behav Immun Health*. 2022;**20**:100412. *https://doi.org/10.1016/j.bbih.2022.100412.*

8.16 Managing anosmia in Long Covid

The anosmia that is specific to Long Covid can be very persistent. It is caused by damage by the virus to the cells supporting the olfactory nerves (sustentacular cells and olfactory epithelial cells), which become infected because they express the ACE2 receptor, to which the virus binds. This increases the production of transmembrane serine protease 2 (TMPRSS2) which promotes virus uptake. It has also been suggested that the virus enters the brain via the olfactory nerve. The damage to the sense of smell can be long-lasting.

At present, there is no definitive treatment. Smell retraining using persistent sniffing of potent smells such as eucalyptus oil, oil of cloves, lemon oil, and rose has been shown to be effective but is slow. It is most effective if begun early. There are no significant side effects. Topical steroids by nasal spray (mometasone furoate) or drops (betamethasone) have not been shown to have anything other than limited benefit. Oral steroids have also been used in combination with olfactory retraining and may be beneficial. The combination of nasal fluticasone spray with triamcinolone paste was slightly more effective.

Other approaches tried include insulin patches, caffeine, minocycline (apparently it reduces olfactory sensory neuron apoptosis) and melatonin, which has olfactory neuron protective effects in a rat model.

At present, the most practical options appear to be olfactory retraining, together with a trial of nasal fluticasone spray. Smell retraining kits are available commercially.

FURTHER READING

Khurana K, Singh CV. Management of anosmia in COVID-19: a comprehensive review. *Cureus*. 2022;14(10):e30425. *https://doi.org/10.7759/cureus.30425*.

Meng X, Pan Y. COVID-19 and anosmia: the story so far. *Ear Nose Throat J*. 2024;103(5):NP312–20. *https://doi.org/10.1177/01455613211048998*.

8.17 Managing relapses

As identified in Chapter 6.6, it is crucial that patients with ME/CFS and Long Covid understand about relapses from the time of diagnosis. Relapses can be triggered by an inappropriate increase in activity, increased stress, including inappropriate pressure from employers and unsympathetic family, and intercurrent infections. The appearance of an unexpected relapse for whatever reason can lead to a secondary catastrophization, which will inevitably make all the symptoms much worse than they would be otherwise. Patients need to understand that a relapse doesn't automatically mean that symptoms will revert to the worst they have ever been. Management by supporting therapists should include this reassurance and convey positive information about reinforcing key management steps relating to activity management, rest, sleep patterns, and mindfulness. The re-introduction of symptom diaries for a short period may be valuable to highlight factors contributing to boom and bust. Going back to basics is usually required. Longstanding patients become good at recognizing warning signs and adapting early to prevent excessive symptoms.

Most therapeutic services for ME/CFS and Long Covid offer time-limited interventions and discharge patients once the therapists are happy that they have an appropriate toolkit to manage their condition. Some allow self-re-referral within a fixed time window after discharge. From the perspective of general practice, it is crucial to ensure that a patient presenting with an apparent relapse of previously stable ME/CFS or Long Covid has not developed any new medical condition to account for worsening symptoms, if necessary, undertaking fresh tests (see Chapter 3.3), rather than simply assume that it is a relapse. If there is no evidence of any alternative new pathology, then it may be appropriate to re-refer the patient back to the therapy service for review. Emphasizing the need to follow guidelines on activity management is essential pending review.

The ME Association has published an excellent guide to managing relapses (see Chapter 6.6 and Chapter 14.1).

8.18 Managing the severely ill

UP to 25% of patients suffer from severe long-term illness due to ME/CFS, according to studies in several countries, and we shall probably see similar outcomes in Long Covid. These patients are housebound or even bed-bound by their symptoms. The severity of post-exertional malaise (PEM) seems to be a predictor of this outcome. This group also tend to have more marked autonomic features suggestive of POTS. Once this is established then even sitting can provoke a reduction in cerebral blood flow, meaning that standard tilt-table testing for autonomic dysfunction becomes impossible and also accounts for the difficulties that they have in moving from being recumbent in a bed to semi-upright in a chair. The current NICE Guideline 206 for ME/CFS has specific advice on the management of the severely ill.[4]

Severely affected patients will be housebound with a limited capacity for activities of daily living and will be dependent on family or carers. If they are able to leave the house, a wheelchair will be required. PEM is severe. The most severely affected will be bed-bound, with very marked sensory intolerance and will be completely dependent on carers. They frequently need to stay in a darkened, quiet room. Eating and drinking is a struggle (due to problems with taste and smell and muscle weakness), and supplementary feeding via NG tube, PEG, or intravenously may be necessary. Speech can be affected. There is generalized pain, often with very marked hyperalgesia, even to light touch, which makes care very difficult. Even quiet sounds, subdued light, and normal smells/odours are not tolerated. There is marked cognitive dysfunction and marked sleep disturbance, with disturbed sleep/wake cycles. Headaches can be troubling. Gastrointestinal disturbance can include nausea, abdominal pain, and food intolerances. Total care is required.

Being bed-bound, with nutritional difficulties leads to other complications, such as severe constipation, progressive osteoporosis (no sun exposure and inadequate diet), pressure sores, respiratory infections, and marked muscular deconditioning, all of which exacerbate the disability and make care more challenging. Secondary depression is marked.

This group of patients frequently falls out of the healthcare net: they do not get to GP appointments and cannot get to hospital. Assessment can be challenging as few medical specialists have adequate time resources to complete a full domiciliary assessment. Planned attendance by ambulance to a dedicated facility may be possible, but the ambulance service can rarely commit to delivering a patient at a specific time when the facilities and doctor are free, nor collecting them at an agreed time after the assessment. Such assessments are much slower than normal clinic assessments, as the patient will tire rapidly. For GPs faced with a long-term severely ill patient, prior discussion with the appropriate regional

---

[4] See section 1.17 of NICE guideline [NG206] Recommendations | Myalgic encephalomyelitis (or encephalopathy)/chronic fatigue syndrome: diagnosis and management | Guidance | NICE.

specialist is strongly advised. Telephone follow-up is possible, but not always adequate. Video consultation can be helpful for follow-up but obviously has serious limitations for initial assessment as no examination is possible. The NHS does not have facilities in most regions for inpatient admission, assessment, and initiation of management, nor does it have adequate therapy support for regular domiciliary therapy. Patients who fall into this group do not do well on general medical or rehabilitation wards as they are invariably noise and bright light intolerant and find normal ward routine a struggle. Domiciliary therapy from physiotherapists and occupational therapists under the NHS is minimal or absent in most circumstances, although where it can be provided then it can be extremely valuable and can lead to significant improvement. Malnutrition and dehydration may be very real risks if patients are unable to feed and drink without assistance. Malnutrition leading to secondary fatigue-inducing deficiencies of key vitamins and minerals may occur. If supplementary feeding is required input of a gastroenterologist for insertion of a fine-bore nasogastric tube or placement of a PEG device may be required. Involvement of an experienced dietician is required.

This group of patients often miss out on benefits as they are too exhausted to go through the application processes, may lack specialist assistance to help with applications, may not be able to access the required medical evidence and may not get adequate social care support in the community. Where high-quality care is provided at home, the results can sometimes be surprising. The use of beds with tilt and sitting facilities means that autonomic dysfunction can be addressed by gradually incrementing the head-up legs-down position. Management of these patients is therefore a long-term therapy challenge that the NHS cannot reliably meet at present. Some support is provided by local and national ME charities, but their resources are limited. Dedicated inpatient rehabilitation facilities are minimal or in most regions non-existent in the NHS. Admission to standard rehabilitation wards tends not to go well for reasons outlined earlier but may be necessary to deal with nutritional problems. Where admission is necessary, it is important that there is an agreed (written) plan outlining the goals for the admission, the assessment, investigation, and treatment with all parties (patient and family, medical staff, therapy staff and if necessary social services) before admission. It is essential that plans for discharge and follow-up are also agreed with all parties *before* admission. This applies particularly if the patient is admitted to a distant supraregional unit. The patient's local hospital may need to agree to admit the patient for step-down care after discharge from the distant supraregional unit if the patient cannot go straight home.

Emergency admission of patients with severe ME/CFS (and Long Covid) is frequently disastrous but may be required. Most A&E Departments in the UK and medical admissions units are staffed by doctors and nurses with no knowledge or experience of managing patients with these conditions. Frequently the patient is labelled as having Munchausen's syndrome or other psychiatric illness, especially if duty psychiatrists are summoned: the organic neurological nature of the illness is not understood. Such patients will have severe sensory intolerance: intolerant to noise, light, smells, taste, and touch, and need to be nursed in a quiet, dim environment. Special beds will be required for comfort. All staff interacting with the patient should receive instruction on the nature of the illness and appropriate management strategies. Three tragic cases occurred in 2024 (see Preface). In one of these cases (Maeve Boothby O'Neill), death was directly attributable to complications of ME/CFS and the death is being investigated by the local coroner. Evidence reported at the inquest has heard that the Trust in question was not equipped to deal with her case and that the Trust's own expert on ME was over-ruled when he identified an appropriate ward for her (see: Fiona Hamilton, 'Killed by ME, the terrible illness that divides doctors', *The Times* Saturday 27th July 2024, pp. 14–15). Medical witnesses at the inquest confirmed that they had had no training in managing severe ME/CFS and that the hospital was not equipped to manage such patients. In this case the coroner, for the first time in a death due to ME/CFS, has issued a 'Prevention of future deaths report', which will be sent to NHS managers and health ministers. The medical director for the Trust Hospitals involved gave evidence that he had approached the NHS's Specialist Commissioning body about the lack of any facility anywhere in the NHS for the inpatient care of the severely ill but was told that ME/CFS was not considered appropriate for its focus! The Medical Director of NHS England, Sir Stephen Powis, noted the deficiency in service but did not indicate any action to remedy it. A junior health minister pledged improvements in research and attitudes. It remains to be seen whether anything useful will result from the promises to do better.[5]

Another patient, Edina Slayter-Engelsman from Scotland also died in 2024, having travelled to The Netherlands, where euthanasia and assisted suicide are legal under strict controls, to end her life. After extensive psychological and psychiatric investigations as well as assessment by an ME/CFS clinic in Amsterdam, it was concluded that there were no other treatment options and her life was ended by lethal injection. She had extreme symptoms, particularly sensory intolerance, and was bed-bound and unable to care for herself.[6]

Following the case of Maeve Boothby O'Neill, there have been more news cases of severely affected patients with ME/CFS left without adequate care, especially in regard to nutrition.[7] These cases again reveal that patients were told that the illness was 'all in the head', confirming the urgent need for proper education about the true nature of the illness.

It is important for doctors to recognize that ME/CFS (and probably in due course Long Covid) can be a severe illness that can lead to death. Empathic holistic care is essential, but this must be based on the correct understanding of the cause of the illness and not on spurious psychiatric diagnoses. All therapists and carers need to be given clear written information about the nature of the illness.

[5] See news article by Fiona Hamilton, 'Coroner's landmark ruling on ME', *The Times*, Saturday 28th September 2024, p. 13.

[6] Lisa Summers, 'There is no help – final message of woman with ME', *BBC News*, 29th July 2024.

[7] Philippa Roxby and Smitha Mundasad, 'I'm too tired to chew food but still can't get care for my ME', *BBC News*, 13th October 2024.

CHAPTER 8

The review by Montoya (2021) gives very clear guidance on the nature and management of severe ME/CFS and should be shared with therapists. It includes a valuable list of ADLs and modifications to consider.

Children with severe ME/CFS provide an even greater challenge, particularly if ME/CFS is misdiagnosed as a psychiatric or functional disorder. Even severely affected children can make good recoveries provided that they receive appropriate supportive therapy at home from both paediatricians and therapists who are knowledgeable about ME/CFS. The paper by Royston et al. (2024) outlines the deficiencies in the care of severely affected children, particularly the lack of domiciliary support. The principles of management outlined in the paper by Montoya will apply to children as well.

FURTHER READING

McDermott C, Al Haddabi A, Akagi H, Selby M, Cox D, Lewith G. What is the current NHS service provision for patients severely affected by chronic fatigue syndrome/myalgic encephalomyelitis? A national scoping exercise. *BMJ Open*. 2014;**4**(6):e005083. *https://doi.org/10.1136/bmjopen-2014-005083*.

Montoya JG, Dowell TG, Mooney AE, Dimmock ME, Chu L. Caring for the patient with severe or very severe myalgic encephalomyelitis/chronic fatigue syndrome. *Healthcare (Basel)*. 2021;**9**(10):1331. *https://doi.org/10.3390/healthcare9101331*.

Royston AP, Burge S, Idini I, Brigden A, Pike KC. Management of severe ME/CFS in children and young people in the UK: a British Paediatric Surveillance Unit study. *BMJ Paediatr Open*. 2024;**8**(1):e002436. *https://doi.org/10.1136/bmjpo-2023-002436*.

Strassheim V, Newton JL, Collins T. Experiences of living with severe chronic fatigue syndrome/myalgic encephalomyelitis. *Healthcare*. 2021;**9**:168. *https://doi.org/10.3390/healthcare9020168*.

Friedman KJ, Bateman L, Meirleir KL de. *ME/CFS—the severely and very severely affected. Healthcare*, special issue on long-term severely affected in 2020 for further articles including articles on children. *https://www.mdpi.com/journal/healthcare/special_issues/me_cfs_issue*.

What drug treatments are available?

9.1 Principles of drug therapy for fatigue

The lack of any immediately obvious drug therapy for ME/CFS has meant that almost all known drugs have been tried at some point! Most have not been shown to be of benefit so far or inadequate clinical trials have been done to confirm benefit. The use of drugs falls into two areas: the use of drugs to 'cure' the illness and the use of drugs to ameliorate symptoms. Doctors often feel under pressure to do 'something', which usually involves reaching for the prescription pad. My experience over the years has been that most of the things that I have tried have not been helpful and in the long term often make patients feel worse from side effects. The MEpedia has a huge list of potential treatments, for most of which it is difficult to see any obvious scientific rationale.[1] Likewise, the current list of trials of treatments for Long Covid include some speculative drugs (Scheibenbogen et al., 2023) for a list of some of the drug trials. However, more science is now

---

[1] MEpedia *https://me-pedia.org/wiki/Category:Potential_treatments*

being applied and novel approaches to therapy are being considered (see 'Further reading').

An important factor in the use of drug therapy of any type is that ME/CFS patients tolerate drug therapies poorly, especially psychoactive drugs, and are more likely to have significant side effects. Trials of drug treatment should therefore start with the smallest possible dose to assess tolerance, followed by slow escalation to assess benefit and side effects. One would expect the same intolerance to apply to drug use in Long Covid.

However, the pressure created by Long Covid has led to more fundamental research and this in turn has led to new ideas for symptomatic treatments although nothing so far suggestive of a curative treatment. As this is now a moving field it is important to keep abreast of potential new therapies. As with much other research on both ME/CFS and Long Covid, treatment studies are often underpowered and/or have other methodological flaws, although this is improving.

Another major issue with drug treatments is that if the media get wind of anything even slightly positive in terms of drug trial results, then the findings get blown out of all proportion. The best (worst!) example of this was the use of rituximab (see section 9.8). This can lead to huge pressure to prescribe, even when the data is only preliminary and has not been confirmed in secondary independent studies.

It is essential that doctors understand everything that the patient is taking, including things they buy over the counter (OTC) or on the internet and check for any potential interactions or side effects. Patients may be reluctant to admit that they are buying unprescribed medications, so direct questioning is required, in a non-judgemental way. Clearly patients do it because they want to try anything that might have a possible beneficial effect and in the absence of any orthodox cures, they can hardly be criticised for this.

Where patients are taking OTC therapies, it is important to make sure that there are no interactions with prescribed medication and that they understand the potential side effects. My own approach has been to encourage patients to undertake their own n = 1 trial by trying the OTC treatment for say 3 months and then stopping and reviewing whether they feel better on or off the treatment. This needs to be a hard-headed assessment, looking for obvious things that have improved on the treatment and have returned once it has stopped. If necessary, the process can be repeated to be certain. This is particularly important when the treatment is expensive. The use of symptom diaries during such trials can be helpful in identifying benefit/absence of benefit.

A recent meta-analysis reviewed the evidence for deficiency of and supplementation with vitamins and minerals and found little evidence to support either major deficiencies or benefits from supplementation. However, many of the studies reviewed were methodologically weak and supplementation studies were often not placebo-controlled (see also section on diet in Chapter 8.13).

CHAPTER 9

FURTHER READING

Novel pharmacological approaches to treatment

Scheibenbogen C, Bellmann-Strobl JT, Heindrich C, et al. Fighting post-COVID and ME/CFS—development of curative therapies. *Front Med (Lausanne)*. 2023;10:1194754. *https://doi.org/10.3389/fmed.2023.1194754*.

Review of drug therapies

Castro-Marrero J, Sáez-Francàs N, Santillo D, Alegre J. Treatment and management of chronic fatigue syndrome/myalgic encephalomyelitis: all roads lead to Rome. *Br J Pharmacol*. 2017;174(5):345–69. *https://doi.org/10.1111/bph.13702*.

Seton KA, Espejo-Oltra JA, Giménez-Orenga K, Haagmans R, Ramadan DJ, Mehlsen J. Advancing research and treatment: an overview of clinical trials in myalgic encephalomyelitis/chronic fatigue syndrome (ME/CFS) and future perspectives. *J Clin Med*. 2024;13(2):325. *https://doi.org/10.3390/jcm13020325*.

Vitamins and minerals

Joustra ML, Minovic I, Janssens KAM, Bakker SJL, Rosmalen JGM. Vitamin and mineral status in chronic fatigue syndrome and fibromyalgia syndrome: a systematic review and meta-analysis. *PLoS ONE*. 2017;12(4):e0176631. *https://doi.org/10.1371/journal.pone.0176631*.

9.2 Anti-viral drugs

Anti-viral drugs, like antibiotics, are quite specific for certain types of viral infections. Unfortunately, many viral infections do not have safe and effective anti-viral drugs. The lack of evidence for a single infection triggering ME/CFS hampers rational use of anti-viral drugs As discussed under causation, it may well be that many different types of infection can trigger prolonged fatigue in susceptible individuals. Viral infections may also act as hit and run agents, leaving behind a disordered immune response, while the triggering virus has long since disappeared. In this setting anti-viral agents will be of no value, unless used in the acute infection. As the definitions of ME/CFS prevent patients being assessed in the earliest stages, it is unlikely that there will be an opportunity to use anti-viral treatments in the initiation phase when there is active viral replication. The use of anti-virals may be of more value in infections where there infections leads to long-term infection, typically with herpesviruses. However, these viruses typical integrate into the DNA and may lie dormant for many years. Anti-virals will therefore be effective only at periods when there is active viral replication. Some viruses may cause chronic infection, but this usually only occurs in patients with very disordered immune systems, for example enteroviruses in certain types of agammaglobulinaemia. The finding of active viral infection in Long Covid is likely to change our view on the use of anti-virals in established ME/CFS and Long Covid, but will need to be targeted against whichever virus is identified.

Because herpesviruses are ubiquitous, many healthy people carry the viruses, which can be reactivated by other viral and bacterial infections or by other illnesses. Defining whether the herpesviruses have a causative role in ME/CFS is therefore difficult and therefore evaluating the role of antiviral agents active against these viruses is also difficult. Some authorities claim that up to 80% of cases of ME/CFS are due to herpesviruses, but the use of specific anti-herpesvirus drugs is less than impressive.

Trials of anti-viral drugs have been largely unconvincing, although it can be argued that the wrong drugs are being given at the wrong point in the illness. Antivirals directed at HSV, EBV, CMV, and HHV6 have all been tried. While aciclovir and derivatives are relative non-toxic, other drugs such as ganciclovir and valganciclovir are much more toxic and should only be used in the context of properly controlled trials by experienced physicians. Benefit has only been observed where there has been evidence of viral infection against which the anti-viral is known to be active. Artesunate, which is active against herpesviruses, was also effective where there was evidence of infection. Antivirals used in the treatment of HIV such as tenofovir and lamivudine have also been tried.

The anti-viral and immunomodulator rintatolimod (Ampligen) has been trialled in ME/CFS, with claimed benefit on cognitive impairment and exercise tolerance, especially where there was evidence of HHV6 infection. It is more probable that any effect is due to immunomodulation rather than an anti-viral effect. Remdesivir has been used as an anti-viral in COVID-19 infection. The antiviral pleconaril, which is active against enteroviruses has also been used, without convincing evidence of benefit.

The problem with the use of anti-virals in ME/CFS is the usual research issue of small trials, lack of placebo control, and high placebo response rates. The lack of clarity about which virus(es) may be triggering ME/CFS and whether these are persistent or transient also impacts treatment selection and the timing of treatment in the course of the illness.

The use of anti-virals early in COVID-19 infection has been associated with a reduction in the risk of developing Long Covid, irrespective of age and vaccination status. The effect has been seen with Paxlovid (a combination of nirmatrelvir and ritonavir) and also with molnupiravir. However, the last drug has been identified as mutagenic, with concern that its use may give rise to new variants of COVID-19 as well as the potential for malignancy. In the Paxlovid trial, treated patients were 26% less likely to develop fatigue at 90 days. Both drugs need to be taken within 5 days of a positive test to be effective, confirming that timing of the use of anti-virals is crucial in preventing fatigue. This is likely to apply to ME/CFS in cases where there is acute onset and a triggering virus is identified but of course almost all patients are seen too late for anti-viral strategies to be effective, especially as the triggering viral event may not be the same in everyone. Whether there is robust evidence for viral persistence in ME/CFS, as has been identified in Long Covid, is also a crucial question that has not yet been answered, although certain authorities have long suspected persistent infection as a contributory factor to pathology in ME/CFS.

The discovery that patients with prolonged post-covid symptoms may have ongoing detectable spike proteins and other proteins, suggestive of continuing viral replication, means that there may be a role for SARS-CoV2 anti-viral therapy after the initial phase. A trial of Paxlovid in Long Covid is underway and will be mapped against long-term viral persistence. Vaccination has been said to improve symptoms. A case report trial of monoclonal antibody therapy using Regeneron (casirivir/imdevimab) showed significant improvement in three patients with confirmed Long Covid (but with poor histories of COVID-19 antibody/antigen status!).

FURTHER READING

Krumholz HM, Sawano M, Bhattacharjee B, et al. The PAX LC trial: a decentralized, phase 2, randomized, double-blind study of nirmatrelvir/ritonavir compared with placebo/ritonavir for Long COVID. *Am J Med.* 2024. *https://doi.org/10.1016/j.amj med.2024.04.030.*

Rasa, S., Nora-Krukle, Z., Henning, N. *et al.* Chronic viral infections in myalgic encephalomyelitis/chronic fatigue syndrome (ME/CFS). *J Transl Med.* 2018;16:268. *https://doi.org/10.1186/s12967-018-1644-y.*

Scheppke KA, Pepe PE, Jui J, et al. Remission of severe forms of long COVID following monoclonal antibody (MCA) infusions: a report of signal index cases and call for targeted research. *Am J Emerg Med.* 2024;75:122–7. *https://doi.org/10.1016/ j.ajem.2023.09.051.*

Strain WD, Sherwood O, Banerjee A, Van der Togt V, Hishmeh L, Rossman J. The impact of COVID vaccination on symptoms of long COVID: an international survey of people with lived experience of long COVID. *Vaccines.* 2022;10(5):652. *https://doi.org/ 10.3390/vaccines10050652.*

9.3 Pain management

Pain in ME/CFS and Long Covid is mainly of the fibromyalgic variety. Occasionally it can be due to other causes such as severe vitamin D deficiency in a patient with restricted sun exposure and inadequate dietary intake. It is therefore important to check that the pain is consistent with FM and that there are no other causes.

Treatment is difficult and the side effects of any drugs tried must be balanced against benefit. Little specific research on the optimum approach to pain management in ME/CFS has been carried out and approaches therefore draw on advice given for the management of fibromyalgia (see section 9.13). Antidepressants, especially tricyclic antidepressants and duloxetine can be tried, along with anti-inflammatories. The latter do not tend to be very effective, as the pain is not generally thought to have an inflammatory origin. Some anti-convulsants can be helpful in managing pain. These include carbamazepine, gabapentin, and pregabalin. All can have significant side effects and can interact with other drugs.

None of these drugs are specifically licensed for use in ME/CFS or Long Covid, although some are licensed for use in fibromyalgia. Most of the drugs have significant side effects.

In the early stages of the illness, most patients are desperate to try anything that might help. Over time, with the realization that the drugs are not curative and have side effects, together with the psychological adaptation to chronic illness which can be facilitated by psychological therapies, many patients reach a point where they would rather live with their symptoms than put up with the side effects of drugs with marginal benefit. Tailing off the drugs slowly is crucial as some drugs (SSRIs and SNRIs) have the potential for significant withdrawal symptoms.

TENS machines may be of some limited value and offer the option of non-drug treatment.

FURTHER READING

Tzadok R, Ablin JN. Current and emerging pharmacotherapy for fibromyalgia. *Pain Res Manage*. 2020;2020. *https://doi.org/10.1155/2020/6541798*.

9.4 Sleep disturbance

ME/CFS and Long Covid are typically associated with sleep disturbance but sleep may also be disturbed by fibromyalgic pain. Sleep is typically unrefreshing, so that patients wake still feeling exhausted. Assessment of the sleep symptoms is a crucial part of the evaluation of a new patient, to ensure that other primary and secondary sleep disorders have been excluded before a diagnosis of a chronic fatigue syndrome is made.

Management of sleep disturbance can be difficult. Proper sleep hygiene is required. Simple steps include the avoidance of alcohol and caffeine for 4 hours before bed, and avoidance of computer/mobile phone/TV use (the blue screen light impairs sleep) before and in bed. A fixed routine of bedtime and getting up is required. While a time-limited nap in the middle of the day is permissible, prolonged periods of sleeping during the day will impair night-time sleep.

Benzodiazepine sleeping medications should be avoided as these have only a short-term benefit and can lead to addiction. Low-dose tricyclic antidepressants tend to work better and are preferred if fibromyalgic pain is a contributor to the sleep disturbance. Sedating anti-histamines can be used as an alternative (chlorphenamine or hydroxyzine). Hangover effects the next morning may limit use.

Melatonin may be helpful. It is recommended for children and older adults but not adults of working age! As tolerance to it develops (due to receptor down-regulation), it should be used for spells of up to 6 weeks followed by a break of a week, which allows the receptors to reset. Some patients find that 5 days on and 2 days off works just as well. As it is not licensed for use in ME/CFS, prescription can be difficult, although, as it is used widely for treating jet lag, it is relatively easy for patients to obtain it over the internet. It is available in both short-acting and long-acting versions. The short-acting versions are best for those who struggle to get off to sleep while the long-acting versions are better for those who struggle to stay asleep. A recent clinical trial has suggested that a combination of melatonin with zinc may be effective. This study used only 1 mg of melatonin, but higher doses may be required.

Melatonin has also been suggested as a theoretical treatment for Long Covid, although not formally trialled yet. Unfortunately, as melatonin has cheap and widely available, there is little incentive for the pharmaceutical industry to support robust clinical trials: these will need to be undertaken by state research funded studies.

FURTHER READING

Cardinali DP, Brown GM, Pandi-Perumal SR. Possible application of melatonin in long COVID. *Biomolecules.* 2022;12(11):1646. *https://doi.org/10.3390/biom12111646.*

Castro-Marrero J, Zaragozá MC, López-Vílchez I, et al. Effect of melatonin plus zinc supplementation on fatigue perception in myalgic encephalomyelitis/chronic fatigue syndrome: a randomized, double-blind, placebo-controlled trial. *Antioxidants (Basel).* 2021;10(7):1010. *https://doi.org/10.3390/antiox10071010.*

9.5 Co-enzyme Q10/NADH

Co-enzyme Q10 (ubiquinone, CoQ10) is a molecule that is important in the normal function of mitochondria. Mitochondrial dysfunction remains an area of interest in the causation of ME/CFS and Long Covid. One study has suggested that levels may be reduced in patients with ME/CFS and that this may be a risk factor for early cardiovascular mortality. There are several small trials of supplementation, either alone or with NADH, which have shown improvements in exercise tolerance, neurocognitive function, and fatigue. This is a supplement that can be readily bought over the counter, although the optimal dose is not yet defined and there are a variety of strengths available (from 30 to 1,200 mg!). Side effects appear to be minimal and include rashes, nausea, heartburn, and diarrhoea. It should not be used with anticoagulants and certain anti-cancer drugs. It does seem to benefit some patients and therefore it may be worth trialling, either alone or with NADH. Neither are prescribable, but can be bought over the counter, with the usual caveat for OTC supplements that they are frequently not standardized and the stated amount on the tablet may be different from the actual content. For neither supplement has the optimal therapeutic dose been identified in proper dose-ranging studies. A large Spanish randomized placebo-controlled double-blind study showing benefit used 200 mg of co-enzyme Q10 with 20 mg of NADH, which obviously gives a starting point for treatment. EUROMENE has indicated that it is supportive of the use of CoQ10 in ME/CFS. Selenium has also been suggested, as an adjunct to CoQ10 therapy.

The role of CoQ10 in Long Covid is uncertain. There have been studies claiming reduced levels of CoQ10 in the mitochondria from platelets in patients with Long Covid. A recent placebo-controlled trial of CoQ10 in Long Covid did not show any benefit, although both the placebo and CoQ10 groups improved over the course of the study! Another small study of CoQ10 with alpha-lipoid acid suggested benefit but this was part of an observational study and not a randomized double-blind trial.

CoQ10 (300 mg/day) has also been suggested to benefit patients with fibromyalgia, with significant reductions in pain. Other studies have suggested a reduction in fatigue, at a dose of 100 mg/day.

Overall, the evidence points towards a probable benefit from CoQ10 in a variety of chronic fatigue-related syndromes. However, there are significant problems with oral bioavailability of CoQ10, which may be as low as 5% in some formulations. This complicates dose-ranging studies and inter-study comparisons.

The abnormalities in the redox state in both ME/CFS and Long Covid have led to the concept of using N-acetylecysteine to alleviate symptoms. Trials are currently ongoing. N-acetylcysteine has been used in acute COVID-19 infection to mitigate endothelial damage. It is also being tested in Long Covid, with the hypothesis that it may reduce cardiac morbidity. It has a range of properties, including blocking various intracellular signalling pathways and regulating cytokine signalling. It has been used for hepatoprotection in paracetamol overdose for many years, so it has the advantage of being well-established. One small trial has used N-acetylcysteine (NAC) in combination with guanfacine, an α2A-adrenoceptor agonist, and shown improvements in cognitive function in Long Covid.

Other anti-oxidants such as ginseng and quercetin have also been suggested to improve fatigue. A randomized controlled trial (RCT) of quercetin showed improved fatigue, sleep, and muscle function.

FURTHER READING

Castro-Marrero J, Segundo MJ, Lacasa M, et al. Effect of dietary coenzyme Q10 plus NADH supplementation on fatigue perception and health-related quality of life in individuals with myalgic encephalomyelitis/chronic fatigue syndrome: a prospective, randomized, double-blind, placebo-controlled trial. *Nutrients*. 2021;13(8):2658. https://doi.org/10.3390/nu13082658.

Fesharaki-Zadeh A, Lowe N, Arnsten AF. Clinical experience with the α2A-adrenoceptor agonist, guanfacine, and N-acetylcysteine for the treatment of cognitive deficits in 'Long-COVID19'. *Neuroimmunol Rep*. 2023;3:100154. https://doi.org/10.1016/j.nerep.2022.100154.

Hansen KS, Mogensen TH, Agergaard J, et al. High-dose coenzyme Q10 therapy versus placebo in patients with post COVID-19 condition: a randomized, phase 2, crossover trial. *Lancet*. 2023;24. https://doi.org/10.1016/j.lanepe.2022.100539.

Mantle D, Hargreaves IP, Domingo JC, Castro-Marrero J. Mitochondrial dysfunction and coenzyme Q10 supplementation in post-viral fatigue syndrome: an overview. *Int J Mol Sci.* 2024;**25**(1):574. *https://doi.org/10.3390/ijms25010574.*

Rondanelli M, Riva A, Petrangolini G, Gasparri C, Perna S. Two-month period of 500 mg lecithin-based delivery form of quercetin daily dietary supplementation counterbalances chronic fatigue symptoms: a double-blind placebo-controlled clinical trial. *Biomed Pharmacother.* 2023;**167**:115453. *https://doi.org/10.1016/j.bio pha.2023.115453.*

9.6 Naltrexone

Low-dose naltrexone, an opioid antagonist, also binds to non-opioid receptors such as TLR4, which is involved in inflammatory pathways. It has been used for the treatment of some chronic inflammatory conditions such as Crohn's disease, multiple sclerosis, and fibromyalgia, where there is significant pain.

It has been suggested for many years to benefit ME/CFS patients when used in low doses. Patients will frequently have read about it and may request prescriptions. *In vitro* studies have suggested that low-dose naltrexone may regulate neuroinflammation and modulate gene activity in NK cells. Unfortunately, the clinical trial data is very limited (one Finnish study between 2010 and 2014) and one more recent mechanistic study *in vitro* in 2021. Not all patients benefit and the side effects of naltrexone can be similar to ME/CFS! A small trial in Long Covid suggested that it was tolerated and might be helpful. Mechanistically there is also a suggestion that naltrexone may interfere with the binding of SARS CoV2 to the ACE2 receptor. It is not currently licensed in the UK or most other countries for the treatment of fatigue conditions.

FURTHER READING

Cabanas H, Muraki K, Eaton-Fitch N, Staines DR, Marshall-Gradisnik S. Potential therapeutic benefit of low dose naltrexone in myalgic encephalomyelitis/chronic fatigue syndrome: role of transient receptor potential melastatin 3 ion channels in pathophysiology and treatment. *Front Immunol.* 2021;**12**:687806. *https://doi.org/10.3389/fimmu.2021.687806.*

Choubey A, Dehury B, Kumar S, Medhi B, Mondal P. Naltrexone a potential therapeutic candidate for COVID-19. *J Biomol Struct Dyn.* 2022;**40**(3):963–70. *https://doi.org/10.1080/07391102.2020.1820379.*

Löhn M, Wirth KJ. Potential pathophysiological role of the ion channel TRPM3 in myalgic encephalomyelitis/chronic fatigue syndrome (ME/CFS) and the therapeutic effect of low-dose naltrexone. *J Trans Med.* 2024;**22**(1):630. *https://doi.org/10.1186/s12 967-024-05412-3.*

Tamariz L, Bast E, Klimas N, Palacio A. Low-dose naltrexone improves post-COVID-19 condition symptoms. *Clin Ther.* 2024;**46**(3):e101–6. *https://doi.org/10.1016/j.clinth era.2023.12.009.*

9.7 Magnesium and other vitamins/minerals/ nutritional supplements

It has been suggested that magnesium deficiency may contribute to muscular weakness and fatigue in ME/CFS, specifically measuring red cell magnesium levels. However, not all studies have confirmed that patients with ME/CFS are deficient in magnesium. Magnesium deficiency is more likely if there is bowel disease that prevents uptake, in vitamin D deficiency and in patients on protein-pump inhibitors. It is worth checking magnesium, calcium and vitamin D levels in patients where muscle symptoms are predominant and/or where sun exposure is limited. Where ME/CFS and Long Covid patients are largely housebound and sun exposure is limited, vitamin D deficiency is not uncommon and appropriate replacement, with mineral supplements, if necessary, may be highly beneficial, improving muscle function and reducing muscle pain.

Magnesium supplementation (either orally or by injection) has been recommended by some practitioners for ME/CFS. Robust clinical trial evidence of benefit is lacking. On the whole magnesium supplementation is safe, although injected magnesium can be painful. Large oral doses of magnesium salts will cause diarrhoea.

Like all therapies, where the evidence base is weak, patients, who do not have evidence of deficiency of magnesium or vitamin but who want to try it should be encouraged to do their own n = 1 trial by treating themselves for a period followed by a period off treatment, to see whether there is really any noticeable benefit. If they cannot identify any improvement, they should be discouraged from continuing to take it on the basis that 'it might help'.

Evidence that deficiency of other vitamins and minerals plays a major role in the causation of ME/CFS is weak. Deficiencies may be secondary (e.g. vitamin D deficiency in housebound patients). Iron deficiency may be a primary cause of fatigue and needs to be treated before a diagnosis of ME/CFS is made. There is some evidence that vitamin E may be low and that supplementation may help. D-ribose, a pentose sugar that is involved in the production of energy in mitochondria is also said to benefit ME/CFS, but robust evidence is lacking. It is thought that it increases energy provision in muscle, especially after exercise. Again, large randomized placebo-controlled trials have not been carried out. It appears to be safe.

While the role of magnesium levels in acute COVID-19 have been studied, there is no evidence for a role of magnesium supplementation in ameliorating symptoms of Long Covid.

FURTHER READING

Bjørklund G, Dadar M, Pen JJ, Chirumbolo S, Aaseth J. Chronic fatigue syndrome (CFS): suggestions for a nutritional treatment in the therapeutic approach (2019). *Biomed Pharmacother.* 2019;109:1000–1007. *https://doi.org/10.1016/j.biopha.2018.10.076.*

Joustra ML, Minovic I, Janssens KAM, Bakker SJL, Rosmalen JGM. Vitamin and mineral status in chronic fatigue syndrome and fibromyalgia syndrome: a systematic review and meta-analysis. *PLoS ONE*. 2017;12(4):e0176631. *https://doi.org/10.1371/journal. pone.0176631*.

Teitelbaum JE, Johnson C, St Cyr J. The use of D-ribose in chronic fatigue syndrome and fibromyalgia: a pilot study. *J Altern Complement Med*. 2006;12(9):857–62. *https://doi.org/ 10.1089/acm.2006.12.857*.

9.8 Immune modifiers

In the late 1980s and early 1990s, the thinking about ME/CFS was that it was likely to be triggered by infection. Coxsackieviruses were part prime suspects (see Chapter 5.3). This was also the time when purified cytokines were being introduced into clinical practice. These included both interferons (alpha and gamma) and interleukin-2. These were tried in ME/CFS, but not only was there no evidence of significant benefit but in some cases symptoms became worse! Because of the complex way the web of cytokines operates, using mega-doses of a single cytokine is unlikely to be helpful. Immune therapies therefore fell out of favour for many years.

The advances in our understanding of the potential role of neuroinflammation and possibly autoimmunity in the generation of ME/CFS and Long Covid has resurrected interest in immunomodulatory therapies. In particular, there is increasing evidence of long-term dysregulation of the immune system, with skewing of immune responses to a Th2 pattern of cytokine production. This provides some potential avenues for immunoregulatory therapies.

Immunoglobulin has been used as replacement therapy in immunodeficient patients since the 1960s, initially as low-dose intramuscular treatment, IMIg. In the 1990s when intravenous preparations became available, higher doses could be used in immunodeficient patients. Both IMIg and IVIg were trialled in ME/CFS but all the immunoglobulin trials in ME/CFS have been either ultra-low-dose IMIg or standard replacement doses of IVIg. There were phases of enthusiasm followed by disillusionment!

A series of trials of IVIg in the 1990s showed no evidence of benefit from IVIg. The usual caveats apply to these trials regarding candidate selection (comparting apples and pears?), as well as the lack of placebo control and blinding. Trial numbers were small, and as noted, placebo responses are very high in ME/CFS. Some of these studies are difficult to interpret because some of the treated patients were identified as having underlying immunological abnormalities (low IgG subclasses) as well as infections, meaning that it is not clear whether these are fatigued patients with primary ME/CFS and minor immunological abnormalities or secondary fatigue due to an underlying primary immunodeficiency.

Despite this, some private practitioners continued to use very low-dose IMIg. The doses administered in IMIg treatment of ME/CFS have been very low and it is difficult to assign any likely benefit. This treatment was never subjected to rigorous placebo-controlled trials. Manufacture of IMIg was phased out by most companies in favour of IVIg, with the exception of specific IMIgs for treating tetanus, rabies, etc. There were small number of chronically symptomatic ME/CFS patients who have claimed that the long-term IMIg was highly beneficial, although provided that they are supported through withdrawal there is no evidence that withdrawal made a significant difference to their baseline symptoms.

More recently, the question of the benefit of IVIg has been resurrected in a review of the previous data from the 1990s by Brownlie & Speight. However, as noted, none of the early trials could be deemed as entirely satisfactory, and reanalysis of such trials does not necessarily make them better. Further trials of IVIg, in conjunction with anti-virals have been carried out in Italy in a cohort of 741 patients, with claims of benefit from the combination treatment. IVIg has also been used acutely in severe COVID-19 infection, with benefit, but also in post-covid patients.

Through the 1990s, evidence accumulated that a number of autoimmune-based diseases could be ameliorated by high-dose IVIg. The possibility of an auto-immune brain component and the presence of autoantibodies (to β2-adrenergic receptor and M3 cholinergic receptors) in ME/CFS does suggest that high-dose IVIg might be beneficial, as in other well-established autoimmune diseases. This would be in immunoregulatory doses rather than the replacement doses used in the older studies. There is still insufficient data to justify routine use of IVIg in either replacement or immunosuppressive doses in ME/CFS, but it is an area that needs to be revisited with properly planned studies with appropriately powered studies blinded and with placebo arms. So far, no trials of immunomodulatory dose IVIg have been carried out in ME/CFS.

Apheresis and immunoadsorption have been used in a few cases of ME/CFS where autoantibodies have been detected, with claimed benefit, and in Long Covid as a putative treatment for 'microclots' (see Chapter 5.8). Further studies of immunoadsorption are ongoing (NCT0510770), which is a randomized double-blinded sham-controlled study. No result has been reported yet.

Immunoglobulin products are derived from donated plasma. In the past there have been a number of outbreaks of hepatitis C associated with the use of immunoglobulin products. All products now marketed are required to have at least two anti-viral steps incorporated into the manufacturing process, active against a prescribed range of model viruses. Donors are required to undergo more stringent testing, and donated plasma is quarantined until the donor is retested at their next donation. Nonetheless immunoglobulin, as a human-derived product, cannot be assumed to be safe, as new blood borne infections may occur which evade the current safety measures. They should only be used where there is clear evidence of benefit and where patients are made aware of the potential long-term risks.

The monoclonal antibody rituximab, directed against the CD20 molecule on B lymphocytes, was originally introduced as a treatment for tumours arising from CD20+ lymphocytes. It is a potent immunosuppressive agent and significant long-term immunosuppression may result from its use in cancer therapy. A Norwegian group identified that fatigue was markedly improved in patients with lymphoma treated with rituximab and tried it in a small cohort of patients with ME/CFS, with apparent benefit. This small open and uncontrolled trial was widely reported, with the effect that clinicians around the world were besieged by patients demanding rituximab. Unfortunately, several follow-up controlled studies showed no evidence of benefit, but these took time to organize and execute. In the intervening period doctors were accused of denying life-changing therapy to ME/CFS patients, with patients saying that refusal to prescribe was based on cost issues, rather than the toxicity and lack of proper evidence. Doctors were rightly cautious about using a potentially highly toxic drug, which causes severe immunosuppression, without strong supporting evidence. This episode demonstrates the difficulties of treatment in this field where there are no curative treatments and should act as a caution about the release of very preliminary data, until follow-up trials have been carried out.

The anti-viral and immunomodulator rintatolimod (Ampligen) has been trialled in ME/CFS, with claimed significant benefit, particularly in energy levels and cognitive function. This drug is said to have both antiviral and immunomodulatory effects, due to the stimulation of the production of interferons. However, despite the trials, it has not yet been granted approval by the FDA for the treatment of ME/CFS.

Treatment of ME/CFS patients who subsequently developed malignancies and were treated with regimes including cyclophosphamide showed improvement in their fatigue. As well as being an anti-cancer drug, cyclophosphamide in lower doses is used as a potent immunomodulatory drug. This has led to small open trials of the use of cyclophosphamide in long-term ME/CFS patients. This showed benefit in over 50%, with some long-term responses. However, as with rituximab, the initial trial did not include a placebo arm, so further studies with a double-blind placebo-controlled format will be required to assess whether cyclophosphamide has a role in the management of patients with ME/CFS. Cyclophosphamide requires careful monitoring for bone marrow suppression and increases the risk of bladder cancer, the risk of which is related to the total cumulative dose. The risk of bladder cancer can be mitigated by the use of mesna.

The role of immune modulators ion Long Covid specifically has not been systematically investigated. The use of a range of immune modulators have been studied in severe acute COVID-19, with the aim of improving outcomes and function. Severity of the initial infection is a risk factor for Long Covid.

FURTHER READING

Brownlie H, Speight N. Back to the future? Immunoglobulin therapy for myalgic encephalomyelitis/chronic fatigue syndrome. *Healthcare (Basel)*. 2021;9(11):1546. *https://doi.org/10.3390/healthcare9111546*.

Fluge Ø, Rekeland IG, Lien K, et al. B-lymphocyte depletion in patients with myalgic encephalomyelitis/chronic fatigue syndrome: a randomized, double-blind, placebo-controlled trial. *Ann Intern Med.* 2019;170(9):585–93. *https://doi.org/0.7326/M18-1451.*

Rekeland IG, Fosså A, Lande A, et al. Intravenous cyclophosphamide in myalgic encephalomyelitis/chronic fatigue syndrome. an open-label phase II study. *Front Med (Lausanne).* 2020;7:162. *https://doi.org/10.3389/fmed.2020.00162.*

Strayer DR, Young D, Mitchell WM. Effect of disease duration in a randomized phase III trial of rintatolimod, an immune modulator for myalgic encephalomyelitis/chronic fatigue syndrome. *PLoS One.* 2020;15(10):e0240403. *https://doi.org/10.1371/journal.pone.0240403.*

Tirelli U, Lleshi A, Berretta M, Spina M, Talamini R, Giacalone A. Treatment of 741 Italian patients with chronic fatigue syndrome. *Eur Rev Med Pharmacol Sci.* 2013;17(21):2847–52. *https://www.europeanreview.org/article/5782.*

9.9 CBD oil

CBD (cannabidiol) oil is derived from cannabis plants (usually grown for hemp rather than for high levels of tetrahydrocannabinol, which is a highly psychoactive drug). CBD oil does not contain tetrahydrocannabinol (THC) and so can be sold over the counter in the UK (although it is banned in some countries and some states in the USA). There is no standardization, so products from different manufacturers can vary widely in effectiveness. It is available as capsules and oil and can be taken orally or sublingually. CBD oil has been shown to be of benefit to some patients with ME/CFS, but there are no controlled trials confirming significant benefit. CBD oil has been shown to act on dopamine receptors and to influence the microglia in the brain, both of which may be highly relevant in ME/CFS and Long Covid. It comprises a number of different chemicals and which ones might be relevant to treating ME/CFS are unknown as yet. The body makes its own cannabis-like substances (endocannabinoids) and therefore has brain receptors for these compounds (which is why cannabis has such an effect). How this impacts on CFS/ME is not known. It is however an anxiolytic. Benefit has also been described in fibromyalgia.

Because CBD oil doesn't have THC in it, there is little potential for addiction and side effects seems to be minimal: occasional reports of abnormal liver function tests, low blood pressure and dizziness, drowsiness, and an increase in Parkinsonian symptoms. The latter may be valuable, as early Parkinson's disease is one of the differential diagnoses for the cause of of chronic fatigue in the older population. High levels are thought to suppress the immune system, although whether this effect is involved in any benefit in ME/CFS is unknown.

A small trial has been undertaken of CBD derivatives in Long Covid with demonstrated benefit, although the trial was unblinded and not placebo-controlled.

Trials have been undertaken with cannabis flowers, which have also shown benefit in fatigue, although the effect was quite variable from patient to patient.

On the whole the lack of evidence of harm suggests that patients may wish to try it, although how beneficial it is must await proper clinical trials.

FURTHER READING

Khurshid H, Qureshi IA, Jahan N, Went TR, Sultan W, Sapkota A, Alfonso M. A systematic review of fibromyalgia and recent advancements in treatment: is medicinal cannabis a new hope? *Cureus*. 2021;13(8):e17332. *https://doi.org/10.7759/cureus.17332*.

Thurgur H, Lynskey M, Schlag AK, Croser C, Nutt DJ, Iveson E. Feasibility of a cannabidiol (CBD)-dominant cannabis-based medicinal product (CBMP) for the treatment of Long COVID symptoms: a single arm open-label feasibility trial. *Br J Clin Pharmacol*. 2023;90(4):1081–93. *https://doi.org/10.1111/bcp.15988*.

Xiaoxue Li, Diviant JP, Stith SS, et al. Vigil; the effects of consuming *Cannabis* flower for treatment of fatigue. *Med Cannabis Cannabinoids*. 2022;5(1):76–84. *https://doi.org/10.1159/000524057*.

9.10 Use of anti-depressants

Often the first approach from doctors to a patient with prolonged fatigue is to consider depression and offer antidepressants. As discussed in the chapter on causation, functional MRI studies of the brain indicate that depression and ME/CFS are different. Anti-depressants are therefore not curative therapies for ME/CFS. However, many patients with ME/CFS become depressed over time because of the impact of their illness on their life. It is important to recognize and treat this secondary depression. The role of anti-depressants, along with psychological therapies is to assist in coping with the consequences of the illness and thereby improve the chances of recovery. No antidepressants have licences specifically for ME/CFS, although some have licences for use in fibromyalgia.

Where anti-depressants are being used to deal with secondary depression consequent upon chronic illness, it is essential that the patient understands that this is likely to be a short-term measure. A review date and end date need to be identified at the start of therapy. Long-term repeat prescription is unhelpful. Most long-term ME/CFS patients find the side effects of the drugs worse than the illness over time and are keen to come off them, which helps.

The selection of anti-depressants to use in this setting will be determined by the prescriber's familiarity with this family of drugs. There is no single anti-depressant that works well. Patients with ME/CFS tolerate psychoactive drugs poorly, so it is important to start with small doses and work up slowly. If one drug is not tolerated, then it is worth trying a different drug.

Older tricyclic antidepressants (tricyclics, TCAs: amitriptyline, imipramine, nortriptyline) can be very helpful, as they may assist in pain management and help improve night-time sleep. However, they can cause daytime sedation, which impacts on fatigue, and have anti-cholinergic side effects such as dry eyes and mouth. Treatment should start with very small doses (10 mg amitriptyline) and escalate gradually as tolerated until there is either benefit or side effects become intolerable. TCAs can be helpful for fibromyalgia, especially at night.

SSRIs (selective serotonin reuptake inhibitors) are often used, usually fluoxetine or sertraline. Personal experience suggests that these tend not to be well-tolerated in ME/CFS, and I have found that citalopram or escitalopram tend to be better tolerated. These drugs do not have a great benefit for pain. SNRIs (selective noradrenaline re-uptake inhibitors) are an alternative, and some are licensed for use in fibromyalgia. Duloxetine is the best known. Venlafaxine can also be used. Both of these classes of drugs can be associated with the acute serotonin syndrome, which may be triggered by the use of other drugs: prescribed (anti-coagulants), over-the-counter (anti-inflammatories) and recreational, as well as some food supplements. Caution needs to be taken when using SSRIs with ginseng, St. John's Wort, 5-HTP, Syrian rue, nutmeg, and foods rich in tryptophan (chicken, turkey, soy, eggs, pumpkin seeds, peanuts, and strong cheese). Severe serotonin syndrome can lead to rhabdomyolysis. There is an increased suicide risk from SSRIs, especially in young people under the age of 25. Other idiosyncratic psychological symptoms can occur. The drugs can also be associated with withdrawal syndrome if the drugs are stopped suddenly, so withdrawal should be a phased, gradual withdrawal over weeks.

FURTHER READING

Castro-Marrero J, Sáez-Francàs N, Santillo D, Alegre J. Treatment and management of chronic fatigue syndrome/myalgic encephalomyelitis: all roads lead to Rome. *Br J Pharmacol.* 2017;174:345–69. *https://doi.org/10.1111/bph.13702.*

Pae C-U, Marks DM, Patkar AA, Masand P, Luyten P, Serretti P. Pharmacological treatment of chronic fatigue syndrome: focusing on the role of antidepressants. *Exp Opin Pharmacother.* 2009;10(10):1561–70. *https://doi.org/10.1517/14656560902988510.*

9.11 Curcumin and other nutraceuticals

Curcumin is the active ingredient in turmeric, which has a long history of use in Ayurvedic medicine as a treatment for inflammation. It can be helpful in arthritis. Although there are small studies suggesting benefits in ME/CFS and fibromyalgia, meaningful clinical trials are lacking. It is usually compounded with black pepper, which is said to improve the uptake of the curcumin. While generally safe (it is a major ingredient of Asian cookery!), there have been reports of liver damage when very high doses have been taken. Benefits have been shown in a murine model of fatigue. At present there is insufficient evidence to recommend it as a routine treatment for ME/CFS. Dosage in OTC preparations is confusing and there are no dose-ranging studies to evaluate any benefit.

A range of other nutraceuticals have been tried in the context of post-viral chronic fatigue ME/CFS and Long Covid. These include elderberry, green tea (epigallocatechin gallate) and, resveratrol (a naturally occurring polyphenol), quercetin (see section 9.5). The scientific evidence to support these agents is limited.

FURTHER READING

Evans JM, Luby R, Lukaczer D, et al. The functional medicine approach to COVID-19: virus-specific nutraceutical and botanical agents. *Integr Med (Encinitas).* 2020;19(Suppl 1):34–42.

Gupta A, Vij G, Sharma S, Tirkey N, Rishi P, Chopra K. Curcumin, a polyphenolic antioxidant, attenuates chronic fatigue syndrome in murine water immersion stress model. *Immunobiology.* 2009;214(1):33–9.

9.12 Corticosteroids and other hormonal treatments

The putative involvement of the hypothalamic-pituitary-adrenal axis (HPA) in chronic fatigue obviously led to trials of corticosteroid replacement therapy (i.e. low-dose hydrocortisone either alone or with fludrocortisone). Crossover placebo-controlled trials showed no evidence of benefit, using clinical scoring of symptoms. Large doses of prednisolone also do not appear to help which is interesting in the context of ME/CFS potentially being a disease of neuroinflammation. However, any steroid-responsive element to the illness may well be early in the course of the illness.

As might be expected, steroids have been used in acute COVID-19 to treat complications. The acute use has been possibly associated with longer-term harm. Corticosteroids have been trialled in Long Covid with a suggestion of benefit, although with the usual caveats about small numbers and lack of blinding and placebo controls. The benefit appeared to be mostly for breathlessness.

Reductions in sex hormones (testosterone and oestrogen) have also led to empiric treatment with replacement therapy, with no obvious benefit. It is likely that the reductions seen in sex hormones are a secondary phenomenon. There have been no satisfactory controlled trials of sex hormone replacement in ME/CFS.

Because of the concept that standard thyroid function tests are inaccurate, there was a vogue for empathic treatment of ME/CFS with thyroxine or unstandardized thyroid extracts (Armour). Some patients did indeed feel better on these regimes. Endocrinologists have however documented risks from the inappropriate use of thyroid hormones, including the risks of exacerbating damage to the heart, through the generation of persistent tachycardia. Formal trials of replacement therapy have taken place in fibromyalgia, but not in ME/CFS. Much of the published evidence is anecdotal. As noted earlier, the potential involvement of the hypothalamus in the neuroinflammatory process means that endocrine abnormalities cannot be excluded but are likely to be secondary. Further robust clinical trials are required to assess the potential for benefit from thyroid hormone replacement and to identify which patients may benefit.

Obviously, there are some patients presenting as chronic fatigue who turn out to have underlying thyroid disease (both over or underactive thyroid), for whom treatment with either thyroid replacement and/or drugs to reduce thyroid overactivity is entirely appropriate. It is also possible that patients with known ME/CFS or Long Covid may develop thyroid disease, unrelated to these diagnoses, as thyroid disease is common. Repeating thyroid function tests may therefore be appropriate, bearing in mind the possibility of thyroid function being abnormal because of concurrent other illness (sick euthyroid syndrome). Where there is doubt about thyroid status, discussion with a thyroid expert is advised.

FURTHER READING

Akter F, Araf Y, Hosen MJ. Corticosteroids for COVID-19: worth it or not? *Mol Biol Rep.* 2022;**49**(1):567–76. *https://doi.org/10.1007/s11033-021-06793-0.*

Blockmans D, Persoons P, Van Houdenhove B, Lejeune M, Bobbaers H. Combination therapy with hydrocortisone and fludrocortisone does not improve symptoms in chronic fatigue syndrome: a randomized, placebo-controlled, double-blind, crossover study. *Am J Med.* 2003;**114**(9):736–41. *https://doi.org/10.1016/S0002-9343(03)00182-7.*

Goel N, Goyal N, Nagaraja R, Kumar R. Systemic corticosteroids for management of 'Long Covid': an evaluation after 3 months of treatment. *Monaldi Arch Chest Dis.* 2022;**92**(2). *https://doi.org/10.4081/monaldi.2021.1981.*

Thomas N, Gurvich C, Huang K, Gooley PR, Armstrong CW. The underlying sex differences in neuroendocrine adaptations relevant to myalgic encephalomyelitis chronic fatigue syndrome. *Front Neuroendocrinol.* 2022;**66**:100995. *https://doi.org/10.1016/j.yfrne.2022.100995.*

9.13 Metformin

It has been found that the oral hypoglycaemic agent, metformin, may reduce the severity of COVID-19 infection and risk of death and may also reduce the likelihood of the development of Long Covid. As well as its anti-diabetic properties, metformin modulates the activity of the PI3K/AKT/mTOR signalling network by targeting AMP-activated protein kinase (AMPK). Via these pathways it regulates both macrophage and regulatory T cell (Treg) function and is thus able to modulate inflammatory immune responses to the virus. At present the evidence on metformin as therapy is largely observational and theoretical and no large-scale trials have been undertaken. The drug has a long history of use in the treatment of diabetes and polycystic ovarian syndrome (PCOS), although there has been recent concern about contaminants in some long-acting formulations, which is being investigated by the FDA.

FURTHER READING

Ibrahim S, Lowe JR, Bramante CT, et al. Metformin and COVID-19: focused review of mechanisms and current literature suggesting benefit. *Front Endocrinol.* 2021;**12**:587801. *https://doi.org/10.3389/fendo.2021.587801.*

Kamyshnyi O, Matskevych V, Lenchuk T, Strilbytska O, Storey K, Lushchak O. Metformin to decrease COVID-19 severity and mortality: molecular mechanisms and therapeutic potential. *Biomed Pharmacother.* 2021;144:112230. *https://doi.org/10.1016/j.bio pha.2021.112230.*

9.14 Treatment of POTS

POTS symptoms in the context of ME/CFS and Long Covid can add significantly to the disability, as they make standing and mobilization much more difficult/impossible. Simple measures should be started first, including ensuring adequate hydration, use of compression stockings, and avoidance of excessive horizontal rest. Blocking the head of the bed on bricks (4–6 inches) helps maintain a degree of lower limb dependency that will help maintain normal postural reflexes. In more severe cases, the use of a fully tilting bed will help. Large meals, excess alcohol, and heat exposure will make symptoms worse, so should be avoided. Special exercise programmes are available to counteract the effects of POTS. Recumbent exercise will help maintain muscular fitness.

If these are not dealing with symptoms adequately, then drug therapy should be considered, but this should be instigated by a physician experienced in the management of POTS and after appropriate confirmatory tests. This can include the use of a non-selective beta-blocker (not in asthmatics) or ivabradine, which interferes with sinus node function to reduce heart rate. Fludrocortisone can be used to increase blood volume, but potassium levels should be monitored and if necessary supplemented. Long-term use can be associated with myocardial fibrosis from chronically raised aldosterone levels. Midodrine, an $\alpha1$-adrenergic receptor agonist, can be effective (not licensed for this use) and should only be prescribed by a specialist.

FURTHER READING

Vasavada AM, Verma D, Sheggari V, et al. Choices and challenges with drug therapy in postural orthostatic tachycardia syndrome: a systematic review. *Cureus.* 2023;15(5):e38887. *https://doi.org/10.7759/cureus.38887.*

9.15 Treatment of fibromyalgia

The diagnosis of fibromyalgia is dependent on a number of criteria, including widespread pain in multiple regions, intrusive fatigue, hypersensitivity to noise, light, temperature (very similar to ME/CFS), and symptoms for more than three months. The Royal College of Physicians (RCP) has produced useful diagnostic criteria with valuable information sheets for patients and doctors.[2] As well as pain, there are typically multiple tender points. Validated self-assessment scoring systems are available (Fibromyalgia Survey Questionnaire).

---

[2] For more information, see the Royal College of Physicians website: *https://www.rcplondon.ac.uk/gui delines-policy/diagnosis-fibromyalgia-syndrome*

Treatment Guidelines were reviewed by EULAR in 2016 and include the use of cognitive behavioural therapy (CBT) or more in-depth psychotherapy for associated depression and anxiety. Recommendations for the management of pain include duloxetine, pregabalin, tramadol (with or without paracetamol); and low-dose amitriptyline or pregabalin are recommended for night-time (see also section 9.10). The use of opiates is not recommended as they tend not to be effective in this type of pain. In the UK, the management of fibromyalgia is covered within the scope of the NICE Guideline on Chronic Pain.[3] However, drug treatment is often not terribly successful and patients may decide that the side effects of the drugs are worse than the symptoms, so with support from psychologists it may be reasonable to phase out ineffective drugs. The RCP has produced some useful handouts for patients as well as doctors.

As discussed in section 9.5, there is some evidence that CoQ10 may be of benefit in fibromyalgia, both for pain and fatigue, with the caveats outlined in that section.

FURTHER READING

Berwick R, Barker C, Goebel A; guideline development group. The diagnosis of fibromyalgia syndrome. *Clin Med (Lond)*. 2022;**22**(6):570–4. *https://doi.org/10.7861/clin med.2022-0402*.

Häuser W, Jung E, Erbslöh-Möller B, et al. Validation of the fibromyalgia survey questionnaire within a cross-sectional survey. *PLoS One*. 2012;**7**(5):e37504. *https://doi. org/10.1371/journal.pone.0037504*.

Macfarlane GJ, Kronisch C, Dean LE, et al. EULAR revised recommendations for the management of fibromyalgia. *Ann Rheum Dis*. 2017;**76**(2):318–28. *https://doi.org/ 10.1136/annrheumdis-2016-209724*.

Wolfe F, Clauw DJ, Fitzcharles M-A, et al. The American College of Rheumatology preliminary diagnostic criteria for fibromyalgia and measurement of symptom severity. *Arthritis Care Res*. 2010;**62**:600–10. *https://doi.org/10.1002/acr.20140*.

9.16 Treatment of irritable bowel and bladder syndromes

Irritable bowel syndrome (IBS) is an almost universal accompaniment to ME/CFS and is seen as a complication post-COVID-19 infection. Symptoms can be very troublesome and can range from minor to severe. As with all bowel symptoms, if there is evidence of new or worsening symptoms, then all guidelines recommend investigation by a gastroenterologist to exclude alternative diagnoses (inflammatory bowel disease, cancer, lactose intolerance, coeliac disease). The basic investigations required for a diagnosis of ME/CFS and Long Covid will exclude many significant conditions (inflammatory markers, Fbc, tTG antibodies) NICE Guidelines for IBS were last updated in 2017.[4] However, the American

---

[3] NICE Guideline NG193 (2021)
[4] *https://www.nice.org.uk/guidance/cg61*

Gastroenterology Association has published more recent (2022) Guidelines for both IBS with predominant constipation and diarrhoea (Chang et al., 2022; Lembo et al., 2022).

Basic management, as recommended in the NICE Guideline cg61, should include:

- Ensuring regular meals and avoiding missing meals or having long gaps between meals.
- Drinking plenty of fluids but avoiding more than three cups of tea/coffee per day
- Reducing or avoiding alcohol, and fizzy drinks.
- Limit intake of high-fibre foods
- Reduce the intake of resistant starch, which is found in reheated or processed foods and which will reach the colon intact
- Limit the amount of fresh fruit
- Avoid the sweetener sorbitol, found in some weight-loss products, sugar-free sweets, and chewing gum
- Use oat-based products with added linseeds for wind and bloating
- Avoid insoluble fibre such as bran
- Trial probiotics
- Consider a low FODMAP (fermentable oligosaccharides, disaccharides, monosaccharides, and polyols) diet—which should only be started under the supervision of a state-registered dietician
- Psychological therapies such as CBT or hypnotherapy may also help.

Pharmacological therapy can include OTC anti-spasmodics, laxatives where constipation is the main issue (ispaghula is best) and loperamide, where diarrhoea is the main feature. Linaclotide is a second-line agent for patients with persistent chronic constipation and where other measures have failed. Tricyclic anti-depressants can used to reduce bowel motility and SSRIs are an alternative, although neither have marketing approval for IBS.

Management of an irritable bladder is less well understood. There is a strong link to IBS. There is overlap with interstitial cystitis, where there is inflammation in the bladder that is not associated with infection. Symptoms include frequent urge to micturate and pelvic pain. Diagnosis, as with IBS, involves the exclusion of other pathologies (infection, prostate in men, gynaecological problems in women) and may require review by a urologist, to undertake cystoscopy and, if necessary, biopsy, renal tract ultrasound, and urodynamic studies. The role of 'allergy' in causation is unproven, although some patients are clear that dietary modification makes a significant difference to their symptoms. Testing for specific IgE to suspect foods invariably gives negative results (skin prick testing and/or RAST testing). Pharmacological treatment depends on the findings of investigation and is complex. Symptoms of frequency can be reduced with drugs such as oxybutynin, solifenacin, and mirabegron. Bladder stretching and instillations may help. A range of other drugs including immunosuppressants are sometimes used for severe interstitial cystitis.

FURTHER READING

Chang KM, Lee MH, Lin HH, Wu SL, Wu HC. Does irritable bowel syndrome increase the risk of interstitial cystitis/bladder pain syndrome? A cohort study of long-term follow-up. *Int Urogynecol J*. 2021;32:1307–12. *https://doi.org/10.1007/s00192-021-04711-3*.

Chang L, Sultan S, Lembo A, Verne GN, Smalley W, Heidelbaugh JJ. AGA clinical practice guideline on the pharmacological management of irritable bowel syndrome with constipation. *Gastroenterology*. 2022;163,(1):118–36. *https://doi.org/10.1053/j.gas tro.2022.04.016*

Colemeadow J, Sahai A, Malde S. Clinical management of bladder pain syndrome/interstitial cystitis: a review on current recommendations and emerging treatment options. *Res Rep Urol*. 2020;12:331–43. *https://doi.org/10.2147/RRU.S238746*.

Homma Y, Akiyama Y, Tomoe H, et al. Clinical guidelines for interstitial cystitis/bladder pain syndrome. *Int J Urol*. 2020;27(7):578–89. *https://doi.org/10.1111/iju.14234*.

Huang KY, Wang FY, Lv M, Ma XX, Tang XD, Lv L. Irritable bowel syndrome: Epidemiology, overlap disorders, pathophysiology and treatment. *World J Gastroenterol*. 2023;29(26):4120–35. *https://doi.org/10.3748/wjg.v29.i26.4120*.

Lembo A, Sultan S, Chang L, Heidelbaugh JJ, Smalley W, Verne GN. AGA clinical practice guideline on the pharmacological management of irritable bowel syndrome with diarrhea. *Gastroenterology*. 2022;163(1):137–51. *https://doi.org/10.1053/j.gas tro.2022.04.017*.

Paramythiotis D, Karlafti E, Didagelos M, et al. Post-COVID-19 and irritable bowel syndrome: a literature review. *Medicina*. 2023;59(11):1961. *https://doi.org/10.3390/medicina59111961*.

9.17 Treatment of other symptoms, including mast cell activation syndrome

Mast cell activation syndrome is a curious condition with symptoms that overlap to an extent with ME/CFS and fibromyalgia. In addition to chronic fatigue, there are repeated episodes of severe allergic reactions (anaphylaxis, generalized hives, acute on chronic bowel symptoms, collapse). During these episodes mast cell markers such as trypatse will be elevated. Consistent triggers are usually absent. There is overlap with idiopathic anaphylaxis. It is distinct from mastocytosis, and there is usually no evidence of excess mast cells either in the skin or bone marrow and certainly no clonal mast cells. In between attacks mast cell mediators are not usually raised. Specific IgE to foods and other allergens are usually absent. It must be distinguished from histamine intolerance, where patients are unusually sensitive to ingested foods with high histamine levels. The diagnosis is suspected by patients more often than it is clinically proven. Bone marrow examination (including analysis for *c-kit* mutations), skin biopsy, and flow cytometry on peripheral blood may be required to exclude mast cell proliferative conditions. Criteria for the diagnosis have been established and include the presence of symptoms in more than one organ system. However, much looser criteria may also be used, which confuse the diagnostic prognosis. Management can be troublesome as the response to chronic high-dose anti-histamines may be poor. Referral to a consultant Immunologist/Allergist is advised if this diagnosis is suspected.

ME/CFS and Long Covid are associated with a range of other recognized symptoms constellations such as fibromyalgia, irritable (functional) bowel and bladder symptoms (discussed in sections 9.13 and 9.14), chronic pelvic pain, migraine, and functional headache. Drug treatment of these conditions should follow the standard guidelines. However, ME/CFS patients tolerate medication poorly and polypharmacy should be avoided and non-drug strategies used if possible. Problems can arise if a patient is attending multiple clinics. It is crucial therefore that one doctor (either a nominated specialist or the GP) is prepared to take overall ongoing responsibility and undertakes a medication/treatment review at regular intervals. This should involve a discussion with the patient to understand the benefits accruing to each medication and any side effects that are being experienced. Liaison with other specialists may be required. This approach limits the number of medical appointments and ensures that only medication of convincing benefit is continued. If the patient is unsure then agreeing a temporary cessation, followed by a further review is sensible. Just because a patient has been taking a medication for a long while does not mean that it is helpful.

FURTHER READING

Buttgereit T, Gu S, Carneiro-Leão L, Gutsche A, Maurer M, Siebenhaar F. Idiopathic mast cell activation syndrome is more often suspected than diagnosed—a prospective real-life study. *Allergy.* 2022;**77**(9):2794–802. *https://doi.org/10.1111/all.15304.*

Gülen T, Akin C, Bonadonna P, et al. Selecting the right criteria and proper classification to diagnose mast cell activation syndromes: a critical review. *J Allergy Clin Immunol Pract.* 2021;**9**(11):3918–28. *https://doi.org/10.1016/j.jaip.2021.06.011.*

9.18 Other drugs

The MEpedia identifies a huge list of drugs that have been tried or proposed for use in ME/CFS. For Long Covid, the emerging science is leading to more focused ideas for therapeutic intervention. For almost all of them, at the moment, the evidence is mostly theoretical or anecdotal and not backed up by properly powered clinical trials. Since many of these drugs are highly toxic, much clearer evidence of benefit is required before they can be recommended. These days, where almost anything can be ordered over the internet if you know what you are looking for, it is important to caution patients about experimentation without prior discussion with a competent healthcare professional.

As discussed, novel approaches based on new science are being developed all the time, so it is crucial to keep a watch for novel treatments backed up by good science.

FURTHER READING

Akanchise T, Angelova A. Potential of nano-antioxidants and nanomedicine for recovery from neurological disorders linked to long COVID syndrome. *Antioxidants.* 2023;12(2):393. *https://doi.org/10.3390/antiox12020393.*

Barnard RT, Siegel EB. A brief survey of interventional agents intended to treat Long COVID. *Microbiol Aust.* 2024;45(1):22–6. *https://doi.org/10.1071/MA24008.*

CHAPTER 9

CHAPTER 10

Prognosis

KEY POINTS

- Early diagnosis and intervention improve outcomes for ME/CFS and Long Covid.
- A proportion of patients remain long-term disabled, some seriously.
- Long Covid and ME/CFS may both follow a relapsing and remitting course.
- The use of anti-virals such as Paxlovid may alter the prognosis in some Long Covid patients.
- Children and adolescents may have a better prognosis than adults, although data is limited.

10.1 Adults

10.1.1 ME/CFS

Many patients, when given a diagnosis of ME/CFS, automatically assume that the condition will not get better. While it is true that not all patients will recover, the reality is that some will recover completely, the majority will improve, albeit with residual symptoms and some limitations in lifestyle, and a small number will remain significantly disabled long term. For a significant number of patients, the illness will have a lifelong impact, which needs to be recognized by healthcare workers. Many of the outcome studies relate to relatively short periods of follow-up, and some are confounded by the fact that some cases initially diagnosed as ME/CFS developed evidence later of other chronic illnesses to account for their fatigue. Overall figures for recovery range between 1 and 31%, with improvement ranging between 8–67%, over a range of different time periods. This indicates that most patients will have a chronic long-term condition, albeit of varying severity.

A number of factors impact on outcome. Age of onset or sex in the adult range of onset does not seem to impact severity or duration of symptoms. Whether the illness is of sudden or gradual onset does not seem to alter prognosis. Severity of the initial illness is, however, a predictor of outcome. The concomitant presence of fibromyalgia symptoms seems to indicate a worse prognosis. Similarly, the presence of significant hypermobility is also associated with more severe disease. Delayed diagnosis is a significant factor in poorer outcomes. Curiously, children and older age groups seem to do better.

Outcomes are improved by early diagnosis and intervention. Delayed referral to specialist services has a negative impact on outcome. This emphasizes the need for prompt attention and referral in primary care. The most crucial factor is the patient's own mindset in relation to the diagnosis. It is quite clear that those who retain a positive outlook on life do better, compared to those who develop a negative mindset about their illness. Therapeutic input to reinforce this at an early stage is therefore crucial. Outcome is also influenced by activity patterns: 'boom-and-bust' activity patterns lead to persistence of or worsening of symptoms. Early introduction of activity management plans appropriate to the individual are therefore critical. Managing expectations while encouraging appropriate activity is an important and difficult role for the therapist and even more so for the patient. While no studies have addressed the issue, continued therapy and medical input are likely to improve outcomes. Short-term interventions are unlikely to be successful.

For long-term patients, there is evidence that symptoms evolve over time. Fatigue may become less of an issue, while neurocognitive problems may become more marked. Many long-term patients have a relapsing and remitting pattern of illness, often driven by external events and intercurrent infections. However, long-term studies of prognosis and outcome are lacking. Personal experience suggests that the greatest chance for recovery occurs in the first two years after the onset of symptoms.

FURTHER READING

Ghali A, Lacout C, Fortrat J-O, Depres K, Ghali M, Lavigne C. Factors influencing the prognosis of patients with myalgic encephalomyelitis/chronic fatigue syndrome. *Diagnostics*. 2022;12(10):2540. *https://doi.org/10.3390/diagnostics12102540*.

10.1.2 Long Covid

Obviously, long-term studies of Long Covid have not yet been carried out. In the historic epidemic forms of virally induced chronic fatigue, the prognosis appears to have been better than in the sporadic form of ME/CFS most commonly seen now; this gives hope that Long Covid may lead to less very long-term illness. Female sex, severity of initial respiratory illness, and concomitant mental health issues seem to be risk factors for prolonged post-Covid symptoms. Similar findings have been identified in other studies of post-infectious chronic fatigue.

Current studies (see Chapter 4.3) suggest that 18–22% of Long Covid patients will still be symptomatic at 12 months. It will be expected that long-term outcomes will be similar to or perhaps better than ME/CFS. This may be modified if more evidence accumulates to support the use of anti-virals to treat early-stage Long Covid.

Myocarditis is a recognized complication of SARS-CoV2 infection and may contribute to long-term disability in patients with Long Covid. The interaction of SARS CoV2 with the ACE-2 receptor is thought to play a role. Likewise, the persistence of abnormal lung perfusion scans and reduced gas transfer factor will contribute to long-term respiratory disability. Similar findings have not been reported in ME/CFS, although there is evidence of abnormal cardiac and endothelial function.

FURTHER READING

Maglietta G, Diodati F, Puntoni M, Lazzarelli S, Marcomini B, Patrizi L, Caminiti C. Prognostic factors for post-COVID-19 syndrome: a systematic review and meta-analysis. *J Clin Med.* 2022;11(6):1541. *https://doi.org/10.3390/jcm11061541.*

10.2 Children

It is thought that children with ME/CFS have a better prognosis than adults, although the data is limited. Recovery was reported by 4–5 years in one study, although the range was 1–15 years, with 60% recovery by 5 years and 88% by 12 years. However, many of those reporting recovery still modified their activities to preserve health and continued to report symptoms not reported by healthy individuals. This still leaves a proportion of children who remain chronically unwell into adulthood.

It appears that one of the most important factors, reported by those who recovered, in helping them was the effort made to ensure their continued involvement in education and support to achieve their aspirations. Maintaining social connections with peers was deemed very important. Supportive therapists were valuable.

The prognosis for Long Covid in children appears to be better than adults, with substantial numbers recovering within 18 months. However, it is likely that there will be some who remain symptomatic for much longer.

FURTHER READING

Esposito S, Principi N, Azzari C, *et al.* Italian intersociety consensus on management of long covid in children. *Ital J Pediatr.* 2022;48:42. *https://doi.org/10.1186/s13052-022-01233-6.*

Rowe KS. Long-term follow up of young people with chronic fatigue syndrome attending a pediatric outpatient service. *Front Pediatr.* 2019;7(21):21. *https://doi.org/10.3389/fped.2019.00021.*

Ying DU, Zhang J, Wu LJ, Zhang Q, Wang YX. The epidemiology, diagnosis and prognosis of long-COVID. *Biomed Environ Sci.* 2022;35(12):1133–9. *https://doi.org/10.3967/bes2022.143.*

CHAPTER 11

Work, school, university, wheelchairs, and travel

> **KEY POINTS**
>
> - ME/CFS and Long Covid are classed as disabling conditions to which the Equality Act (2010) applies.
> - Adjustments will be required for schooling, university, and employment. These need to be reasonable for both the patient and the employer/institution.
> - The social and mental benefits of remaining in education and work, if possible, are significant.
> - Wheelchairs can widen horizons and prevent patients from becoming housebound.
> - Travel, especially flying, requires careful preparation and extra rest before and after the journey.

11.1 Employment

Employment is a difficult area and every case has to be judged on its own merits, depending on the type of employment, type of contract, etc. The key point is that ME/CFS and now Long Covid are legally accepted as disabilities, so are covered by the Equality Act [2010]. The ME Association has a comprehensive guide to employment issues.[1] This guide also covers ill-health retirement and pensions. Action for ME has a similar document.[2] The Trades Union Congress (TUC) has worryingly reported that two-thirds of patients with Long Covid had experienced unfair treatment at work.[3] All the legal and medical principles outlined in the ME/CFS publications apply just as much to Long Covid. There is also a legal question regarding liability for healthcare workers suffering Long Covid, if adequate personal protective equipment (PPE) was not provided, and mass action by NHS staff (doctors and nurses) is underway, seeking compensation. Case law, through an employment tribunal, has confirmed that Long Covid is classed as a disability in Mr T. Burke vs. Turning Point Scotland.[4]

[1] https://meassociation.org.uk/2024/02/an-essential-guide-to-employment-issues-for-people-with-me-cfs-or-long-covid/
[2] https://www.actionforme.org.uk/uploads/me-and-work.pdf
[3] https://www.tuc.org.uk/research-analysis/reports/workers-experience-long-covid
[4] https://assets.publishing.service.gov.uk/media/62a1feace90e07039e31b82c/Mr_T_Burke_v_Turning_Point_Scotland_-_4112457.2021_-_Preliminary.pdf

In the acute phase, early on, work is clearly not possible. There is often pressure on sufferers to return to work early, which is usually unhelpful as it is inevitably too soon and makes the illness worse. A series of failed returns to work looks worse (from an HR perspective!) than one long period of absence. I always encourage sufferers to engage early with their employer's occupational health service. Occupational health are entitled, with the worker's permission, to seek reports from treating specialists. This requires the person to complete a form of permission, which should include a question about seeing the report before it is sent to the OH department. I always advise that the employee should request to see the report first. This ensures that the employee knows exactly what has been said about them and has the opportunity to correct any factual errors before the report is finalized and sent to their OH department. I also remind patients that the OH department is employed by the company and does not have the same duty of care towards the staff as the treating specialist. They must balance the needs of the company against the individual.

After the acute phase, the next area of contention is when and how a return to work can be organized. This obviously depends largely on what the employee's role is. Returns to work should be done slowly over months, not days or weeks. Too many returns to work fail because the company's idea of a phased return is a couple of weeks on half-time and then back to normal working. This won't work in ME/CFS or Long Covid and risks setting the employee back even further. Redeployment may be required if the job is unsuitable.

Union support is often extremely valuable in the early stages and employees are advised to take a union representative to any meetings with HR, to ensure that due process is being followed. As noted, ME/CFS and Long Covid are classed as chronic and disabling conditions for the purposes of the relevant discrimination law (Equality Act [2010]), so employers have an obligation to make necessary adjustments to working conditions to enable a person with these conditions to continue to work if appropriate. The law is of course vague about exactly what adjustments need to be made as the law cannot specify every single condition and job! There may, therefore, be a gulf between the adjustments that the patient thinks are appropriate and the adjustments that the employer offers. Adjustments must be 'reasonable' and reasonable includes being achievable and not unduly onerous/expensive for the company. Reasonable adjustments might include reduced hours, short working days, options for working from home for some or all of the time, improved disabled access, parking close to the workplace, access to a rest area, being taken off shift working, among others. Occupational health should be advising the company and should seek clarification from the treating specialist/therapist to confirm reasonableness. Problems arise most often in small companies with limited resources. The test of reasonableness takes into consideration the impact on the company as well as the patient.

There will be many ME/CFS and Long Covid sufferers for whom a return to work is not feasible because of the severity of their condition and/or the nature of their job, despite reasonable adjustments. In this case, the next stage will be consideration of retirement on ill-health grounds. This must be supported by both Human Resources and by the employer's occupational health service and will require a detailed report from the treating specialist. See the section on pensions (Chapter 12.4).

11.2 School

My practice did not include children, but I did look after a number of teenagers over the age of 16 who were in the final years of their schooling. Like everything else, schools varied considerably in their response to student disability (of all types, not just ME/CFS or Long Covid!). Because schools tend to be judged on their success in getting students through GCSEs, A levels, and into university, students who struggle with the normal rate of progression are often discouraged or asked to leave. However, studies have shown that schools and schooling are felt to play an important part in their recovery by adolescents. The response of teachers is frequently hampered by a lack of knowledge about the nature of ME/CFS and now Long Covid and how it will affect children and adolescents. Doctors and therapists therefore need to liaise closely with schools and teachers and provide appropriate education and support. This will include detailed clinical letters to the school. ME/CFS charities in the UK have support workers who can advise schools, although they are few in number.

The Department of Education in England has provided general guidance to schools on how children with medical conditions should be handled in schools.[5] The bottom line is that School Governing Boards have a duty to ensure that arrangements are in place to support children with medical conditions and enable them to participate fully, including in school trips and physical education (where this is appropriate). They also have a duty to liaise with health and social care professionals, parents, and pupils to ensure that the needs of children with medical conditions are properly understood and effectively implemented. Where a child has been absent for a period, proper plans for reintegration are required.

The best schools offer amended timetables, accommodate extra years to complete exams and allow part-time attendance with supported home study (hopefully this will be better organized after the experience of general home teaching through the COVID-19 pandemic). They also provide quiet areas for rest and accommodate wheelchairs, which may be necessary to help students get around large campuses.

Affected students are entitled to extra time for examinations. It is possible to insist on a single exam per day with a later start. Schools may resist this because of the complication of invigilation and the need to isolate the student to prevent the sharing of information on the questions by other pupils. However, this approach gives the ME/CFS or Long Covid student the best chance of completing exams

---

[5] Department for Education, Supporting pupils with medical conditions at school (2014) *https://www.gov.uk/government/publications/supporting-pupils-at-school-with-medical-conditions-3*

successfully. Where writing is difficult, it may be possible to use a scribe to write the exam answers to the student's dictation. Letters from the responsible consultant or a knowledgeable GP will be required, and these need to be prescriptive in terms of recommendations.

Where schools are unhelpful, teenagers with chronic fatigue conditions may actually be better served in some sixth-form or higher-education colleges, where there is less emphasis on a one-speed track to exams. Such institutions often have other students who for many reasons, often including health and disability issues, never completed formal education, and the institutions are therefore better at managing inclusivity, whatever the disability.

The biggest problem that disabled students find at school is that they rapidly disengage from most of their peers who usually have no concept of chronic illness (unless they have first-hand experience at home) and are at risk of being bullied for being 'different'. This can lead to school refusal. Wheelchairs can be helpful in maintaining engagement with peers' activities (see section 11.4).

Wherever possible, the emphasis should be on maintaining involvement in mainstream schooling, even if only part-time, rather than defaulting to homeschooling. The latter leads rapidly to social isolation, which is highly damaging to mental health. Evidence from follow-up studies on children with ME/CFS confirms that the best outcomes are achieved where education and social interaction can be maintained and affected pupils encouraged to meet their aspirations.

FURTHER READING

Clery P, Linney C, Parslow R, Starbuck J, Laffan A, Leveret J, Crawley E. The importance of school in the management of myalgic encephalomyelitis/chronic fatigue syndrome (ME/CFS): issues identified by adolescents and their families. *Health Soc Care Commun.* 2022;30(6):e5234–44. *https://doi.org/10.1111/hsc.13942.*

Similä WA, Nøst TH, Helland IB, Rø TB. Factors related to educational adaptations and social life at school experienced by young people with CFS/ME: a qualitative study. *BMJ Open.* 2021;11(11):e051094. *https://doi.org/10.1136/bmjopen-2021-051094.*

11.3 University

There is no reason why higher education should be barred to young people with ME/CFS or Long Covid, and the normal requirement of the Equality Act [2010] applies. However, some universities are very averse to making the necessary adjustments and make it as difficult as possible for disabled students. On the other hand, there are others that go to extraordinary lengths to support their disabled students and ensure that they can complete their courses. Over my working career, there has been a significant improvement in the accessibility of higher education to disabled students. All universities should have an officer responsible for disabled students. ME/CFS and Long Covid patients who are considering which universities to apply to should start the process by talking to the disabled student officer and the course leader. If the response is offhand and unhelpful at this stage, then it is unlikely to be better when the student gets there: applications to alternative institutions are strongly advised, no matter how 'good' the academic record of the first institution. If the response is full and enthusiastic and there is a 'can-do' attitude, then it is likely to work.

It is useful for ME/CFS and Long Covid sufferers to get reports from their specialists, including therapists, which outline their special needs (Chu et al., 2020). This should be submitted early and certainly before starting a course, to ensure that the requirements can be met in full. Some universities will have specific forms for the medical advisers to complete. There is a specific allowance for disabled students (Disabled Students Allowance), and the University's Disability Office should be able to advise how to apply for this. It is usually done through the student finance portal, although if a student loan is not required, it can be applied for as a standalone via a separate form. Disabled Students' Allowance (DSA) is a grant, not a loan, so it doesn't need to be paid back. It can cover additional equipment or living/travel costs because of disability. There will be a specific assessment with specialist advisers who will advise on what will be required. It does not affect the entitlement to other benefits such as PIP.

Typical adjustments that are required might include additional time for assessments and exams (as discussed earlier in section 11.2), the ability to log on to lectures remotely and be able to review them at a slower pace (or to have an amanuensis to take notes if a lecture does not have an online version), the ability to study part-time, on-site quiet residential accommodation, usually ground-floor unless there are lifts, near to sites of lectures/practicals and access to regularly prepared meals if preparing meals is a problem for the student. Taxi fares may be covered by DSA if living at home is better. Letters from specialists and therapists need to be precise in advising the additional requirements, which should be done on an individual basis and in discussion with the student.

Overall, there are no courses that are off-limits. I have had a number of medical students with ME/CFS, all of whom have qualified, although once qualified their working conditions may need significant adjustment to allow them to complete their postgraduate training. The only student who did not complete their course was a dental student, for whom the physical demands of the practical work, carried out from standing prevented her from completing the course. Obviously, the problems do not cease upon qualification as a doctor, and therefore detailed career planning and involvement of the NHS Occupational Health Service before taking up house officer posts or later training posts is crucial to success. Modifications to on-call rotas and/or shift working are essential to prevent relapses.

Courses that require fieldwork or industrial placements need careful thought, but again none are off-limits. All-terrain wheelchairs are useful for fieldwork. Many employers are excellent at coping with disabled students, but arrangements need to be checked out in well in advance. This should be organized by placement supervisors in the university, with detailed liaison with the industrial partner's HR department. The student needs to be directly involved in the discussions to ensure that arrangements are manageable.

FURTHER READING

Chu L, Fuentes LR, Marshall OM, Mirin AA. Environmental accommodations for university students affected by myalgic encephalomyelitis/chronic fatigue syndrome (ME/CFS). *Work*. 2020;**66**(2):315–26. *https://doi.org/10.3233/WOR-203176*.

11.4 Wheelchairs

There is considerable resistance to the use of wheelchairs by patients with ME/CFS, particularly young patients. I am in favour of the careful use of wheelchairs, where it enables the sufferers to engage in activities that would otherwise be impossible; for example, going out shopping, or going out on trips with friends and family. The benefits of normal social activities outside of the home are significant when they are structured to avoid exhaustion (boom and bust). Wheelchairs help with this. Clearly, manual self-propelled wheelchairs are a non-starter. Collapsible wheelchairs that can easily be loaded into the back of a car are ideal for carers to use. I do not support the indiscriminate use of wheelchairs in the house.

Young sufferers often become housebound because they cannot participate in the activities that their peers are doing. Persuading them to have wheelchairs means that they can engage in some activities if they have an empathic friend who will push the chair. As their peers usually have little or no concept of chronic illness and young sufferers with ME/CFS often do not look sick, the use of a wheelchair reinforces to their peers that they are ill and do need help, rather than just that they are odd and don't want to socialize. On a number of occasions, this approach has unlocked significant improvements in mood and functioning, once they realize that they can join in. This applies equally at university. I had one student of geography, who could manage around campus okay, but the field trips were a problem. The use of a wheelchair and the recruitment of able-bodied students to push the chair enabled her to participate successfully in most of the field trips.

The same applies also to more mature adults, where a wheelchair will enable the sufferer to join in with family activities rather than be left at home. This helps re-establish a more normal family dynamic. Encouraging outdoor activity in this way is highly beneficial: it increases natural vitamin D production and exposure to normal daylight outdoors also improves sleep patterns.

The use of electric wheelchairs is more controversial. It can be a huge advantage to the severely affected, again enabling activities out of the house. NHS wheelchair services however always seem to flag up difficulties—can the patient manage the chair safely; might they be prone to blackouts (less likely in a chair than if they are standing up)? Overall, for a few patients who have gone ahead, usually with private purchases, it has been helpful.

Therapists appear to have an intrinsic resistance to the use of wheelchairs, it seems on the grounds that it will stop the sufferer from 'exercising' and that the sufferers will become wheelchair dependent. Both of these suppositions are spurious in my experience. Wheelchairs enable patients to have wider horizons and indeed encourage exercise as they can get to different and more interesting places to exercise. They can go around a huge shopping mall without difficulty, getting out of their chair to look around a shop, and then using it to get to the next one. It provides a safety net, so they know they will be able to get back safely to the car. In most cases, sufferers' resistance to using wheelchairs acts as a natural brake to excessive dependence.

11.5 Travel

Sufferers from ME/CFS and Long Covid should be eligible for a Blue Badge, to enable the use of disabled parking. This requires an application to the local council. Success will be improved with an explanatory letter from the GP or specialist, identifying the nature of the disability. Some patients have received abuse because superficially they do not appear to be 'disabled'. In the case of difficulties, the patient support organizations can offer help. Having a Sunflower Lanyard, designed for those with hidden disabilities, can be helpful.[6] This is widely recognized internationally. Cards can be generic or personalized to state the illness (ME/CFS or Long Covid). The cards have personal details including a photo, brief details of the disability, and details of someone to call in an emergency.

More extensive travel, particularly air travel, is always problematic for patients with ME/CFS and Long Covid. It needs to be planned carefully and well ahead of time. An ME/CFS patient and her partner organized a round-the-world trip, which they referred to as the 'slow trip' over 4 months, so with careful planning almost anything is possible. Healthcare professionals should not discourage patients from travelling, provided that appropriate planning is undertaken. A very useful checklist is provided by ABTA for patients with medical conditions and disabilities, which should be completed in advance and shared with the travel agent/tour operator/airline, etc., at booking and before travelling.[7] Extensive general advice is also available on the UK Government Website.[8]

Flying requires very careful planning. Firstly, the patient should explore which airlines have the best record of handling people with disabilities, or conversely which have terrible reputations (usually but not always budget airlines). Using scheduled flights tends to be safer, although more expensive. Patients should check with the airline customer service about support. Even if wheelchairs are not routinely used, some airports are so large that a wheelchair is strongly advised to

---

[6] *https://hdsunflower.com/uk/shop.html*
[7] *https://www.abta.com/sites/default/files/media/document/uploads/Checklist%20for%20disabled%20and%20less%20mobile%20passengers%2010042018.pdf*
[8] *https://www.gov.uk/government/publications/disabled-travellers/disability-and-travel-abroad*

get from check-in to the boarding gate. This may be booked through the airline or through the airport operator. This needs to be done for both departure and arrival airports and for outbound and return. It is important to get written or email confirmation of the booking. Where the patient is already a wheelchair user, the patient should insist that their wheelchair is loaded into the cabin and not just put in the hold, or if it is in the hold, it is loaded so it can be accessed first on arrival.

I always advise patients to have 24–48 hours rest before leaving and on arrival, to allow for recovery. Planning holiday activities needs to be done carefully, allowing plenty of rest time between activities. Patients with postural orthostatic tachycardia syndrome (POTS) particularly should be reminded to increase their fluid intake if the holiday is somewhere hot.

Holiday health insurance is an absolute must. Most travel policies bought through travel agents exclude pre-existing conditions or impose unreasonable loadings. There are however companies who specialize in travel insurance for those with disabilities or pre-existing illnesses. An internet search will identify a range of companies, and patients should be advised to shop around. AllClear is one such company.

Doctors and other specialist healthcare therapists should provide patients who are travelling with clear letters confirming the diagnosis, degree of disability and any medication and their contact number in case healthcare is required away from home and providers need additional information. Any special requirements need to be spelt out, such as wheelchair transfers in airports.

Patients must travel with up-to-date prescriptions indicating which medications they are taking. Customs and Immigration in some countries are very strict about bringing in medication. It is essential that medication is in the packaging in which it was dispensed. The same applies for any over-the-counter medication. It may be advisable to check customs requirements before travelling.

CHAPTER 11

CHAPTER 12

Benefits and pensions

KEY POINTS

- Navigating the benefit system is very difficult for patients with chronic fatigue.
- Many patients do not receive the benefits to which they are entitled.
- Assistance from patient organizations is valuable in ensuring successful application and dealing with appeals.
- Unions are often helpful in dealing with ill-health retirement, which can be complex.
- Despite medical advances confirming the medical nature of the illnesses, the incorrect perception of ME/CFS and Long Covid as psychosomatic or factitious illnesses increases the difficulty in accessing benefits, pensions, and insurance.

12.1 Introduction to benefits

One of the biggest areas of difficulty for people who suffer from ME/CFS and now Long Covid is that of benefits and related issues such as pensions and insurance. While matters have improved significantly, for most of my time working in the fatigue service, there was institutional prejudice against ME/CFS, based on the narrative that the illness was psychiatric or psychological rather than a medical illness. The lack of any reliable biomarkers of 'illness' made it difficult for sufferers to 'prove' their ill-health and therefore, when they inevitably lost their jobs due to ill-health, getting any type of benefit was impossible. Assessors for the Department of Work and Pensions (DWP) were uninformed about the illness and produced inappropriate reports. Insurance companies followed the same line. Even after the publication of a range of expert reports confirming that ME/CFS was a real medical illness, it took a long time before perceptions in the DWP and the Insurance industry changed. The insistence that the diagnosis be confirmed by a hospital specialist increased the workload of my clinic substantially, often with longstanding patients where the diagnosis had already been clearly established and there was no change that would merit medical reinvestigation. A large part of my time was spent preparing medical reports for outside agencies, none of whom paid either me or the NHS for the considerable additional work, which was not clinically indicated. The system also placed the responsibility for obtaining any supporting reports on the patient, rather than directly seeking reports. This hurdle just increased the stress and anxiety in patients already stressed and anxious as a result of a chronic life-changing illness.

Agencies rarely accepted reports from specialist ME/CFS therapists, even though they were often better placed than I was to assess a person's functional capacity. I therefore developed a functional assessment screening tool, based on the DWP questions but with scope for the person to provide their own words, which was far more useful than a simple tick box (see Chapter 14.2). Because benefits are often time-limited, reviews were required before each renewal. Such reviews are driven by administrative rather than true clinical need and are time-consuming. Whether this constituted a valid use of a scarce specialized clinical resource is debatable. It is certainly one way in which one Government Department increases the costs and inefficiency of another!

More recently there is evidence that DWP is ensuring that those to whom it contracts the medical assessments are better briefed on ME/CFS. However, the individual assessors are not always fully familiar with the latest information. Face-to-face assessments are extremely stressful for patients with ME/CFS and Long Covid, particularly those with severe disease, who have word-finding and concentration difficulties. I always advise that patients should ensure that they have a witness present throughout the assessment to record the questions asked and the answers given, as occasionally the assessment reports submitted bear no relation to the patient's recollection of their responses to the questions. Ideally, the witness should not be a close relative but an independent friend, so that collusion between two family members cannot be argued. However, having a relative present is better than not having a witness at all. The friend or relative should make it clear to the assessor at the start that they will be taking notes of the assessment. If there is no witness, it will be the assessor's version that is accepted, not the patient's. If there is an independent witness, then it is easier to challenge any assessment. Independent witnesses can also ensure that a vulnerable patient is not harassed into making untrue statements.

The self-help appendix (Chapter 14.1) includes the details of organizations such as Disability Rights UK, which can provide information and assistance.

12.2 ESA, PIP, and Universal Credit

The benefits system is byzantine in its complexity and it is certainly not designed to be easy for a sick person to navigate, particularly if they have cognitive problems. Many patients give up trying to apply or apply without really knowing the ground rules and are therefore rejected. This makes their illness harder to manage. The majority of people who have become ill with ME/CFS or Long Covid have been in employment and have paid both taxes and National Insurance. There is an assumption that when they require help it will be given automatically but sadly this is not always the case. Many people who have been in employment may have little or no idea about the benefits system: what they are potentially eligible for and how to apply. As well as state benefits there may also be Local Authority benefits such as housing benefit and modification of homes to make them fit for use by people with disabilities. There may be grants available from charities too.

There is of course a political dimension: Governments of all persuasions are always wanting to minimize the expenditure on benefits and to be seen to get 'shirkers' back to work. The bottom line is therefore to pay as little as possible for the shortest time to the fewest people. It is easy to see that patients with ME/CFS and Long Covid are going to be an easy target because there is no current diagnostic test and the prevalent attitude is that it is not a 'real' disease. This means that sufferers have an Everest-sized mountain to climb to get benefits that they are entitled to. The important message to patients is do not give up if you are refused.

The greatest success is achieved if applicants get help from organizations that are familiar with the system and how to complete the forms. The relevant patient support organizations (see Chapter 14.1) can advise to a degree and some have benefits specialists. Citizens Advice Bureaus are also able to advise. However, Government has slashed the budget for these and therefore the level of help is lower (another way in which citizens are disempowered from receiving advice about how to deal with Government and large corporations).

It is essential, for success, to have a medical report. There was a phase where the DWP would only accept medical reports on ME/CFS from medical consultants specializing in ME/CFS and would not accept reports from General Practitioners. This meant that patients would not get benefits until they had been reviewed by a consultant. This added a further time constraint: a referral had to be made from general practice and then there would be a wait to see the consultant. Latterly reports from other specialist therapists seem to be acceptable.

Most people when filling in the benefits forms want to present themselves in the best light or are reluctant to admit to themselves just how disabled they are, but this is counter-productive and can be a major reason for rejection. These forms are about what the patient cannot do and what their illness is like on their worst days.

12.3 Appeals and tribunals

If an application for benefits has been refused by the DWP, then the first stage of challenging the decision is to request a mandatory reconsideration. The decision will be reviewed internally by a more senior person in the DWP and will be based on the evidence submitted. It is essential therefore that the initial submission needs to be an accurate reflection of how bad the illness is and to have an appropriate supporting letter from a healthcare professional. There is a time limit after the initial decision for a request for a mandatory reconsideration (the details will be in the decision letter).

If this too is rejected, then the next stage is to appeal the decision to a tribunal. The tribunal system is separate from the DWP and is part of the Department of Justice. The tribunal will consist of a judge (as chairman), assisted by a professional adviser (often a retired doctor) and a layperson. Yet more forms will have to be filled in, and again getting help with this is essential. As time may have passed since the original submission, it may be advisable to get an updated medical report. Other supportive information can be submitted but patients should be advised not to submit every single download from the internet that they can find on ME/CFS or Long Covid: this does not impress the tribunal and may even be counter-productive. The focus of the submission should be on how the illness affects the patient, with examples, and include well-argued statements about why the initial decision by the DWP was incorrect. This is where having an independent witness to the DWP medical assessment is invaluable. If necessary, the friend's transcript of the assessment should be submitted, where this is at odds with the medical assessor' report.

Applications to tribunals can be either a paper only submission, where the applicant and the DWP simply submit their paperwork and there is no require-ment for either side to appear in person. This is superficially attractive to people with ME/CFS for whom an oral hearing would be very challenging. However, the success rate for paper only as opposed to in person appeals is much less. So the advice is always for the patient to be prepared to appear in person. It is also es-sential for them to take to take a friend or helper, or even better someone familiar with the system from a support organization. The DWP rarely if ever appears in person at tribunal hearings. The tribunals will consider the evidence and are able to come to a completely different conclusion to the DWP, based on the same evidence. Overall, there is a high success rate for appeals (over 60%).

If the tribunal rules against the patient, then it is possible to request that the de-cision be set aside or to appeal the verdict to the upper tribunal (administrative), which can be done on grounds that the tribunal did not give adequate reasons for its decision or that it did not apply the law correctly. In both cases, formal legal advice about how to proceed is required. The decision letter from the tribunal will give detailed information on the process of challenging the decision. Appeals to the upper tribunal are eligible for legal aid.

The decision processes are slightly different in the other home nations in the UK. The processes are accessible through the Home Nations' administrative websites.

12.4 Pensions

A question that crops up regularly concerns early retirement on grounds of ill-health. Like Benefits applications this can be a difficult process. How to approach it depends entirely on who operates the pension scheme, as all the schemes have different rules. For large companies, referral for consideration of early retirement on health grounds is usually initiated by the employee in discussion with human resources (HR) and occupational health. HR must make the referral to the pen-sion scheme and will normally base the decision on a report from Occupational Health, who should have requested a specialist report from the treating clinicians and therapists. The best employers will often to be able to fast-track therapy support privately through Occupational Health. If this is offered, it should be accepted as not to do so will prejudice any subsequent application for ill-health retirement.

Almost every pension scheme is slightly different. If a ME/CFS or Long Covid sufferer is a member of a union, then they will usually have pension advisers who are familiar with the different company schemes and can support the patient through the process. In this setting it is important that patients do not to ditch union membership as soon as they are not able to work, as support will usually only be available to current members.

The age at which the person with ME/CFS or Long Covid becomes ill will largely determine the outcome. The closer to the official age at which a pension can be taken within the scheme, the easier the process becomes. The clinician looking after the patient must be able to make a statement that they do not believe that the person will recover before the normal pensionable age. The longer the gap, the harder it is to predict the future! The other quirk of pensions is to establish whether the ill-health retirement is based on an 'all work' or 'own job' criterion. Incapacity for 'All work' is obviously harder to prove for the future than 'own job'. This has implications also for the person undertaking limited paid work later if there is some improvement. This would be permissible if the pension was awarded on the basis of inability to do their own job, but not if the pension is awarded on the basis of incapability to do any work. Usually, the pension provider's in-house retained medical adviser will review the evidence submitted but Pension Trustees may require an independent medical review in addition to reports from the treating physicians and therapists. Depending on the independent medical adviser's views on ME/CFS, the reports may need to be challenged.

Some pension schemes will offer a partial ill-health retirement pension for a fixed period with a requirement for a medical review. If the illness persists or worsens, then the pension will be upgraded to a full pension. The pension offered will be determined by the length of service and/or contributions.

If there are problems with a private pension scheme then there should be an appeal process and, if this fails, then the other option is to make an application to the Financial Services Ombudsman for a ruling (a slow process but free) or to consider legal action (expensive).

The state pension in the UK is only claimable when reaching the prescribed age. It is calculated on the basis of National Insurance contributions. If the patient is receiving Employment Support Allowance (ESA), then this will pay the NI contributions. However, PIP does not pay contributions, so if a patient is on this benefit, or are receiving a private ill-health retirement pension, it will be worth exploring whether they should be paying additional NI contributions to make up the number of years to the minimum required to get a full state pension. At least 10 years of contributions are required to get any state pension and 35 years to get the maximum. If a patient is not on an indefinite PIP award prior to State pension age, then it is important to ensure that it is renewed for a term that will last until that age is reached. When the State pension age is reached, PIP will be converted into an indefinite award (in practice still reviewed every 10 years!). It is possible to apply for increased benefits under PIP if the patient's needs change, for example mobility. Receiving PIP does not reduce state pension benefits. ESA ceases when you start receiving the state pension.

12.5 Insurance companies

Patients with CFS/ME and Long Covid may encounter problems with Insurance Companies, for example over critical illness insurance. Some can be as obstructive and unhelpful as official bodies. One patient reported to me that his insurance company had set up surveillance outside his house to prove that he could go out and was therefore fit for work, even though his 15-minute slow walk (encouraged by me) was followed by spending the rest of the day resting in his house. The surveillance report recorded his walking out, but not how long he walked for and whether he went out again. He made a complaint to the Insurance Ombudsman, with appropriate medical reports, and won.

Insurance companies may also commission reports from other (paid) experts, generally those who take a line that is supportive of the insurers' position, rather than truly independent or with relevant specialty expertise. These have in the past usually been those supporting the view that ME/CFS is a psychological disorder or form of somatization. Detailed reports from a physician familiar with the evidence that ME/CFS and now Long Covid are recognized *medical* conditions are usually required to overturn these external reports. Additional reports from therapists may be required, as well as reports on functional capacity.

CHAPTER 13

Conclusions

KEY POINTS

- Long Covid and ME/CFS form part of the spectrum of chronic fatigue conditions, with a shared aetiology involving most likely involving neuroinflammation.
- Further research is required in ME/CFS to look for possible persistent virus infection, using modern tools, in the light of finding in Long Covid.
- Current paradigms of ME/CFS need to be updated to remove the focus on the illness as purely psychological and/or psychosomatic.
- More healthcare investment is required to improve knowledge and skills and to provide access to care and benefits for patients, especially the severely affected.
- The UK Government Interim Delivery Plan on ME/CFS (2022–2024) addresses research, attitudes, and education, and living with ME/CFS. Whether, in the light on the critical state of the NHS, this will lead to change remains uncertain.

13.1 Conclusions

Initially Long Covid was treated as a different condition from ME/CFS but with the passage of time it is now clear that these represent the same illness and probably form part of a larger spectrum of post-infective chronic fatigue syndromes. While Long Covid initially has been easier to diagnose than ME/CFS, this will become harder with the passage of time, as more people have evidence of past infection with COVID-19 and/or have been vaccinated. The withdrawal of widespread community screening programmes means that more and more patients with Long Covid will simply present as 'chronic fatigue'. The differential diagnosis of chronic fatigue is covered in some depth in Chapter 3 and this remains important to ensure that other treatable conditions causing chronic fatigue are identified.

Thanks to SARS-CoV2 and the development of Long Covid, we are now seeing high-quality science which is applicable to ME/CFS and is confirming that both conditions are recognizable chronic medical, not psychosomatic or psychiatric illnesses. The science is now focussing on both conditions having the same underlying neuroinflammatory processes, although many other biological abnormalities are being identified (see Chapter 5). The concept of persistence of SARS-CoV2 virus as a potential driver of neuroinflammation in Long Covid and the association of other persistent viruses with post-acute syndromes means that it is important to search for persistent virus in cerebrospinal fluid (CSF) and/or brain tissue in patients with ME/CFS as well. Retrospective application of modern tests for identification of active infection to cases of longstanding ME/CFS are required. It is now clear that past paradigms of ME/CFS as a hysterical, psychosomatic or psychiatric disorder are entirely inappropriate and inconsistent with the current understanding of the science underlying the condition.

The advances in the understanding of the physiology of fatigue are leading to a more directed approach to the assessment of novel approaches to treatment, but at the time of writing, there have not been any startling breakthroughs in treatment. Therapeutic trials are usually hampered by their small scale and lack of proper placebo control. More consideration of the timing of therapeutic interventions is required to avoid comparing apples with pears.

There is considerable work to be done on changing the perceptions of healthcare staff and officialdom and ensuring that the correct messages about ME/CFS and Long Covid are widely disseminated. Attitudinal change is also required across government agencies dealing with benefits, pension agencies, and insurers.

Most importantly, the NHS needs to improve its care for patients with Long Covid and ME/CFS, recognizing that these are long-term chronic disabling conditions, no different to diabetes or MS, and that short-term approaches do not add value. In particular, the string of news reports in 2024 about poor knowledge and care for patients with ME/CFS in the NHS, including the deaths of several patients, highlights the inadequacies that need to be addressed, in particular in terms of inpatient care for the severely affected, with a need to develop specific dedicated inpatient facilities, run by staff with up-to-date knowledge and skills in regard to ME/CFS and Long Covid. Much more training and education is required.

It is helpful that the UK Government has published an interim delivery plan on ME/CFS in 2024, aimed at improving the quality of care.[1] This has been accompanied by the launch of an online learning module by NHS England.[2] However, this requires an NHS or Athens account to access it. Like all online learning you can provide the water and lead the horses to it, but whether they actually drink is another matter. However it is a start, but the results of implementation will be the measure of success or failure. No clear plan is provided for the care of the severely affected.

---

[1] My full reality: the interim delivery plan on ME/CFS—GOV.UK
[2] ME Association https://meassociation.org.uk/2024/05/nhs-england-launches-new-e-learning-module-on-me-cfs/

Appendices

The resource list and patient function questionnaire can be downloaded by locating the 'end matter' of this title at academic.oup.com: search for '9780198962137'

14.1 Resources for patients with ME/CFS, Long Covid, and associated conditions

This is a list of resources, not just for CFS and Long Covid but for the related problems that are also associated with ME/CFS. These resources should be used in conjunction with—and not instead of—proper medical and therapy care.

Management guides

Fighting fatigue. Sue Pemberton & Catherine Berry. Hammersmith Press London, 2009. This is now available as an eBook.

This is the **essential** self-help guide which covers all the basics of activity management.

The Long Covid self-help guide. From the specialists at the post-Covid clinic, Oxford. Green Tree Bloomsbury Publishing, 2022.

This is a well-written and easy-to-understand self-help guide for Long Covid.

CFS unravelled. Dan Neuffer. Elednura Publishing, 2017 (available on Amazon).

This is an interesting book by an Australian Physicist who has spent a lot of time while recovering from CFS researching the science behind CFS. It has a lot of helpful information and advice but should not be viewed as an alternative to proper medical and therapist care. This does not include the most recent advances consequent on the Covid pandemic and Long Covid. It may be hard-going if you don't have much of a science background! It also covers postural tachycardia syndrome (POTS), fibromyalgia, and multiple chemical sensitivity.

Living with ME and chronic fatigue syndrome. Gerald Coakley & Beverley Knops. Penguin Life Experts, 2022.

This is a recent book which has some useful background, particularly around the science of what may cause ME/CFS, and guidance on how to manage it. It doesn't go into a great deal of depth about alternative management strategies.

The Long Covid handbook. Gez Medinger, Professor Danny Altman. Penguin Health Handbooks, 2022.

This is quite a dense guide to Long Covid, but with a lot of useful science. It is better for gaining an understanding of the condition, but the Oxford clinic's guide is a better source of structured self-help for Long Covid.

> *Classic pacing for a better life with ME. Ingebjørd Midsem Dahl. Writersworld, 2020 (English translation).* Available as eBook for Kindle on Amazon.

This book, written by a patient, has a very detailed practical description of how pacing actually works in real life. Invaluable as a resource. Not necessarily up to date with new science, but it doesn't really affect the main messages.

The following small and inexpensive books published by Amazon UK give useful practical advice on how to manage day-to-day, although these may be out of print currently (look for second hand copies).

> *101 Tips for coping with ME. Guidance from a sufferer. Hayley Green.* Amazon, 2013.
> *150 tips for everyday living with ME/CFS. Anna Cayder.* Amazon, 2013.

The MEpedia is a Wikipedia-like project which has a huge collection of information about ME. It contains a lot of very useful information, written by dedicated volunteers, including experienced scientists and clinicians, although the information is not always balanced. *https://me-pedia.org/wiki/Welcome_to_MEpedia.*

Children with ME/CFS

Action for ME have produced a valuable booklet on ME/CFS in Children:

> *https://meassociation.org.uk/wp-content/uploads/DIAGNOSIS-MANAGEM ENT-IN-YOUNG-PEOPLE-A-PRIMER-JUNE-2017.pdf.*

Dealing with relapses

The ME Association has a useful downloadable guide on the management of relapses in ME/CFS, which will be equally applicable to Long Covid:

> *https://meassociation.org.uk/wp-content/uploads/RELAPSES-EXACERBATI ONS-AND-FLARE-UPS-FEBRUARY-2023.pdf.*

Support

The following organizations provide support and, if necessary, help and advice over benefits.

> National: Action for ME: *https://www.actionforme.org.uk/* or telephone 0117 927 9551; for Welfare Advice, call 0800 138 6544

Supporting research into ME/CFS: ME Research UK. This organization funds high-quality research projects in the UK and elsewhere. You can donate to support research and friends and family can organize fundraising events. The charity produces a regular newsletter giving updates on research, and details of current grants are available on the website.: *http://www.meresea rch.org.uk/*. This site also has a wealth of useful information from patients, carers, professionals, and employers. There is a book on Severe ME by Emily Collingridge advertised to buy on the website, although this seems to be unavailable currently.

The ME Association also has lots of useful information and advice: *https://www.meassociation.org.uk/*.

Both of these organizations also provide support for patients with Long Covid.

Long Covid Support is a UK Charity to help people with Long Covid: *https://www.longcovid.org*. Another organization is Long Covid SOS: *https://www.longcovidsos.org*. The latter has leaflets for GPs and patients.

The Sunflower Lanyard may be a useful way of identifying hidden disability (especially when travelling and in some supermarkets); further information at *https://hdsunflower.com/uk/shop.html* and *https://www.bbc.co.uk/newsround/49345642*. The cards can be personalized with the illness (Long Covid or ME/CFS), a photograph, and a brief description of the disability and emergency contacts.

Benefits

Claiming or renewing benefits is always very stressful. If possible, get assistance from someone familiar with the system. The ME Charities may be able to assist (ME Association and Action for ME). The ME Association provides a series of guides on how to apply for and appeal decisions on PIP—see:

https://meassociation.org.uk/?s=PIP+Guide.

Action for ME provide a downloadable guide, although they ask for donations:

https://www.actionforme.org.uk/uploads/pdfs/PIP-overview-Sep-2022.pdf.

Disability Rights UK also provide very helpful factsheets, including advice on Disabled Students Allowance.

https://www.disabilityrightsuk.org/how-we-can-help/benefits-information/fac tsheets/factsheets-alphabetical-order.

They publish a comprehensive guide to benefits (updated annually but costs £45 + £8 for the updater in 2024): *https://shop.disabilityrightsuk.org/products/dis ability-rights-handbook-2024-2025*. They also publish other very useful guidance books, such as: *https://shop.disabilityrightsuk.org/products/winning-your-benefit-appeal-what-you-need-to-know-5th-edition?srsltid=AfmBOopkTYe4vosZvRDQwSFoRT 269EGfbjLSE76TPtlf6zkzS-lFfdRo.*

CHAPTER 14

Another source of advice is:

> *https://www.moneyhelper.org.uk/en/benefits/problems-with-benefits/where-to-get-help-and-advice-about-benefits.*

This site signposts you to agencies that may be able to assist with benefit problems, including sources of free legal advice.

The sites mentioned here also provide benefit support. Scope UK has a section of its website devoted to Long Covid and benefits: *https://www.scope.org.uk/advice-and-support/long-covid-and-disability-benefits.*

It is important to get update medical reports to accompany your application. DWP no longer request medical reports—it is up to the applicant to get these and send them in with applications. Please ensure that you give your doctors enough warning. Requests for reports to be done by the next day are unlikely to be successful. Consultant reports carry more weight.

Information for employers

Another source of frustration can be the lack of knowledge of the condition by employers. Action for ME have produced a sizeable guide for employers. This can be downloaded at:

> *https://www.actionforme.org.uk/uploads/pdfs/employers-guide-to-me-booklet-2016.pdf.*

There is also a guide for patients in relation to work at:

> *https://www.actionforme.org.uk/uploads/me-and-work.pdf.*

The ME Association has a similar document:

> *https://meassociation.org.uk/wp-content/uploads/2024/09/EMPLOYMENT-ISSUES-FEB-2024.pdf.*

Mindfulness

> *Wherever you go, there you are. Mindfulness meditation for everyday life. Jon Kabat-Zinn. Piatkus Books, 1994.*

This is an introduction to mindful meditation, which is a valuable tool for coping with chronic health issues. It is based on Buddhist meditational principles. However, it is not easy to use the book as an instructional manual audio CDs of a mindfulness course by Jon Kabat-Zinn are available (through Amazon) and are a better way of self-guided study. Look for 'Guided Mindfulness Meditation Series 2' audio CD, as this is the CD that goes with the book. Be warned that the CD has periods of silence (deliberate) during which you are expected to meditate.

An alternative (which comes with its own CD!) is:

> *Mindfulness for health. A practical guide to relieving pain, reducing stress and restoring wellbeing. Vidyamala Burch and Danny Penman. Piatkus Books, 2013.*

A new book looking at Mindfulness-based therapy, including Breathworks, specifically for ME/CFS, and aimed at healthcare practitioners is:

> *McKechnie F. Mindfulness-based therapy for managing fatigue: supporting people with ME/CFS, fibromyalgia and Long Covid. Jessica Kingsley Publishers, 2023.*

Headspace is an app for iPhones and Android phones (as well as computers) that gives a course of sessions for mindfulness: the initial course of 10 sessions is free and you can then buy additional sessions as required:

> *https://www.headspace.com/headspace-meditation-app.*

For the sceptical, the following book gives the background of the hard science behind mindful meditation: it's autobiographical and also easy to read.

> *The emotional life of the brain: how its unique patterns affect the way you think, feel, live—and how to change them. Begley S & Davidson R, 2013.*

Lightning Process

This is a training programme, based around neurolinguistic programming. It was originally used as a business management training tool. The science behind neurolinguistic programming is controversial. It is not currently available in the NHS, although is undergoing trials. It has been used in ME/CFS and some patients have tried it with benefit. It is however expensive to do the course.

The website gives some information: *https://lightningprocess.com/what-is-the-lightning-process/.*

Phil Parker, who developed the programme, has written an introductory book, which explains the process (and which covers chronic fatigue/ME), although it cannot be used as a self-help guide.

> *An introduction to the Lightning Process. The first steps to getting well. Phil Parker. Hay House, 2012.*

This is also available to download from the website as an audiobook.

Chronic pain

All the available evidence currently suggests that almost all drugs used for chronic pain become less effective over time when taken continuously. This includes simple drugs such as paracetamol, codeine, as well as morphine-based drugs and drugs such as gabapentin (and related drugs). In particular, morphine-based drugs should be avoided if possible because they markedly increase central fatigue and increase the risk of falls.

Resources for managing pain can be found at:

http://www.paincd.org.uk/resources.

The British Pain Society has a number of useful advice sheets and a link to 'Opioid Aware' a web-based resource about the use of morphine-based painkillers:

https://www.britishpainsociety.org/british-pain-society-publications/patient-publi cations/.

A useful book is:

You can conquer pain. Leon Chaitow. Watkins Publishing London, 2012.

Another book that is recommended for pain is Mindfulness for Health by Vidyamala Burch & Danny Penman (see section 14.1.7)—this comes with its own CD.

Fibromyalgia

Evidence suggests that powerful painkillers are no more effective for chronic pain than simple painkillers and have the potential to cause harm if taken continuously. Minimizing medication is therefore helpful. Stretching exercises may be helpful and mindful meditation (see earlier) is also helpful.

Fibromyalgia and myofascial pain. A practical guide to getting on with your life. Dr Chris Jenner. A How To Self-Help Guide. Oxford, 2011.

This book is aimed at people with predominant fibromyalgia, but chronic fatigue is usually an element of this condition too, so there is much that is useful to people with chronic fatigue as well.

See: https://www.nhs.uk/conditions/fibromyalgia/ for UK-based guidance and additional links.

The following site has a lot of useful information (American!):

http://www.webmd.com/fibromyalgia/default.htm.

The UK patient support organization is Fibromyalgia Action UK:

http://www.fmauk.org/.

Sleep

Overcoming insomnia and sleep problems. A self-help guide using cognitive behavioural techniques. Colin Espie. Robinson Books, 2010.

For patients with sleep disturbance, the following online resource is extremely valuable and is being used by GPs.

https://sleepstation.org.uk/.

There is an excellent range of resources (video and print) from this site for all types of sleep disorders.

https://sleepstation.org.uk/resources.

Irritable bowel syndrome

This is very common in patients with CFS. Helpful dietary guidelines can be found at:

https://www.bda.uk.com/resource/irritable-bowel-syndrome-diet.html.

Beyond this, there is the FODMAP diet which is much more complicated. It is strongly advised that professional advice is sought before embarking on a low FODMAP diet. The following resources give more detailed information:

https://stanfordhealthcare.org/content/dam/SHC/for-patients-component/ programs-services/clinical-nutrition-services/docs/pdf-lowfodmapdiet.pdf.

http://www.rgal.com/wp-content/uploads/sites/11/2013/11/FODMAP-Diet-Chart.pdf

http://www.ibsdiets.org/fodmap-diet/fodmap-food-list/.

For some menu ideas try:

Low FODMAP menus for irritable bowel syndrome: menus for those on a low FODMAP diet. Suzanne Perazzini, 2014.
The complete low-FODMAP diet. The revolutionary plan for managing symptoms in IBS, Crohn's disease, coeliac disease and other digestive disorders. Dr Sue Shepherd & Dr Peter Gibson, 2014.

or

http://www.taste.com.au/recipes/collections/low+fodmap+diet+recipes.

Postural tachycardia syndrome (POTS)

This is a syndrome of excessive tachycardia (fast heart rate) when standing up, which can make people feel dizzy and faint. It is common in patients with CFS, and may also be accompanied by low blood pressure. Diagnosis is usually made in a Falls & Syncope Service by a test called an 'active stand'. The initial treatment is usually to increase water intake and salt in the diet, but drugs can be used too.
Further information can be found at: *http://www.potsuk.org/.*

CHAPTER 14

Cancer-associated fatigue

Fatigue is very common in association with cancer and the treatment for cancer, but is often overlooked. Usually this resolves promptly within 6–12 months of completing treatment but in a small number of cases, it can persist for years. Long-term fatigue is not explained, and does not seem to relate to how successful the treatment has been. Management involves the same sort of strategies as other types of fatigue, including chronic fatigue syndrome.

Further information can be found at the Macmillan website:

> *https://www.macmillan.org.uk/information-and-support/coping/side-effects-and-symptoms/tiredness.*

This webpage has a downloadable book dedicated to the management of fatigue. Macmillan Cancer Support can also provide access to counselling to help cope with the fatigue (see links on the website).

Alternative therapies

There are many alternative therapies that people have tried. The ME Association has advice about the most commonly used therapies. I recommend you check this out before embarking on other therapies.

> *https://meassociation.org.uk/literature/items/alternative-and-complementary-approaches-to-management/.*

Stress

> *Overcoming stress: a self-help guide using cognitive behavioural techniques. Lee Brosnan & Gillian Todd. Constable & Robinson, 2009.*

Post-traumatic stress disorder (PTSD)

This is a complex area and usually requires specialist psychological input. Basic information can be found at:

> *https://www.rcpsych.ac.uk/mental-health/mental-illnesses-and-mental-health-problems/post-traumatic-stress-disorder.*
> *https://www.nhs.uk/mental-health/conditions/post-traumatic-stress-disorder-ptsd/overview/.*

A very useful introductory guide is:

> *Getting past your past. Francine Shapiro. Rodale Press, 2012.*

This book gives some useful basic self-help techniques based on eye movement desensitization and reprocessing (EMDR), as well as explaining how post-traumatic stress may arise and how it affects people. It is NOT a substitute for proper assessment and treatment.

Medically unexplained symptoms/persistent physical symptoms

The following websites are useful in helping understand symptoms which are real but remain medically unexplained:

> *http://www.rcpsych.ac.uk/healthadvice/problemsdisorders/medicallyunexplai nedsymptoms.aspx.*
> *https://www.nhs.uk/conditions/medically-unexplained-symptoms/.*

The last website is rather limited in advice but links to a lot of other resources

Unexplained neurological symptoms

There is an excellent website for people with unexplained neurological symptoms, which has a wealth of self-help resources to download:

> *http://www.neurosymptoms.org/.*

14.2 **Functional questionnaire**

This questionnaire can be used to gather information on functional impairment relevant to providing supporting letters for patients with ME/CFS or Long Covid. Patients need to be given time to complete this and encouraged to use their own words to describe exactly how the illness affects them. They may need help from a relative or friend. It is also useful tool to monitor changes. Completed forms should be stored in the patient record.

Functional capacity questionnaire for patients with CFS/ME or Long Covid

Please complete the questions that follow. This will give me additional information that will be valuable in the event that you need me to prepare reports for benefits, occupational health, pensions, and insurance. The more information you give the easier it is for me to help you.

Walking

How far can you walk before you need to stop? What stops you walking?

Do you use any aids when walking or going out (stick, frame, wheelchair)? Do you need any help from another person? Specify help required.

Does your house have stairs? Can you climb the stairs? What stops you climbing stairs?

Do you have falls or blackouts/dizzy spells while walking inside or outside?

Activities of daily living

Do you need help to get washed, have a bath, or shower?

Do you need help to go the toilet? Specify help required

Can you prepare and cook a meal for yourself? Do you need help?

Do you need any help with eating (special aids or help from a carer)?

Can you get in and out of bed without help? Specify help required.

Do you need any help to get dressed and undressed? Specify the help required.

Do you have any difficulties during the night? Do you require any assistance during the night? Specify the help required.

Do you need any help with taking your medication (medication box, help from carers, reminders)?

Do you live by yourself? Do you have any regular carers (friends, family, paid carers)? How often do they visit?

Communication/Memory

Do you have problems with communicating with other people? Please specify in what way your communication is affected.

Do you have problems with your memory? Please give examples of how this affects you: for example, leaving baths to overflow, forgetting cooking such that it burns, etc.

Do you need to write lists, use reminders on a mobile phone or use Post-It notes?

Do you need help with your hobbies and/or religion?

Can you manage your own financial affairs? Do you need help from someone else? Please specify the help required.

Can you read books and/or follow films (i.e. concentrate without losing the plot and needing to re-read or re-view or ask someone else what is happening)?

Can you go out and plan a route without getting lost (do you need to take someone with you?). Can you follow a map (either on paper or on an app)?

Any other comments

Do you have any other comments about how ME/CFS or Long Covid affects your lifestyle? Give as much information as you can.

CHAPTER 14

Please return to:

Dr J. Anybody
WellHealth Medical Centre
Any Street
Wherever
Anyshire

Or by email to:

wellhealthpractice@anyprovider.com

Index

For the benefit of digital users, indexed terms that span two pages (e.g., 52–53) may, on occasion, appear on only one of those pages.

As this book is about ME/CFS and Long Covid, occurrences of these terms will not be included in the index, with the exception of definitions.